MERGER TRENDS 2

CAUTION:

Catholic Health Restrictions May Be Hazardous to Your Health

CATHOLICS FOR A FREE CHOICE

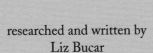

researched and written by
Liz Bucar

ISBN 0-915365-34-0

Trends in Brief

IMPACT OF CATHOLIC/NON-CATHOLIC MERGERS AND AFFILIATIONS

Number of mergers and affiliations between Catholic and non-Catholic hospitals, 1990–1998: 127

Number of mergers and affiliations between Catholic and non-Catholic hospitals, 1998: 43

Number of states that experienced a Catholic/non-Catholic merger or affiliation, 1990–1998: 34

Chances a consolidation eliminated all or some reproductive health services: 1 in 2

CATHOLIC SOLE PROVIDERS

Number of Catholic hospitals which were sole providers in 1997: 76

Number of Catholic sole providers in 1998: 91

Increase in number of Catholic sole providers, 1997–1998: 20%

Percentage of Catholic sole providers in counties with a minority-Catholic population: 95%

CATHOLIC EVER MORE

Number of Catholic hospitals purchased by non-Catholic hospital chains, 1990–1997: 10

Number of Catholic hospitals purchased by non-Catholic hospital chains, 1998: 5

Percentage of sold Catholic hospitals that continue to abide by the *Directives*: 100%

ACCESS TO EMERGENCY CONTRACEPTION

Number of Catholic hospital emergency rooms surveyed by CFFC: 589

Percentage of surveyed hospitals that deny emergency contraception to rape victims: 82%

Percentage of those denying emergency contraception that refused to provide a referral: 31%

All figures are as of January 1, 1999, and are based on mergers and affiliations identified by CFFC.

Table of Contents

Introduction

Since Catholics for a Free Choice first raised questions about how mergers and affiliations of Catholic and non-Catholic hospitals affect access to reproductive health services, we have continued to monitor and report events, analyze trends, and provide information to hospitals, the general public, and advocates of reproductive health services on challenges to these services.

In April 1998 CFFC published *When Catholic and Non-Catholic Hospitals Merge: Reproductive Health Compromised,* which identified serious threats to women's reproductive health services. This report was followed by a six-month review, *Merger Trends: An Update to Reproductive Health Compromised*, analyzing consolidation activities between Catholic and non-Catholic hospitals from January through June of 1998.

Caution: Catholic Health Restrictions May Be Hazardous to Your Health summarizes hospital merger activity in 1998. Included in this report are:

- an explanation of why Catholic/non-Catholic hospital mergers threaten access to reproductive health services;
- documentation of the continuation or curtailment of reproductive health services in Catholic/non-Catholic consolidations in 1998; and
- a close examination of access to emergency contraception—an emerging issue not only in the merger debate but also in Catholic health care—including the results of a CFFC study of the provision of emergency contraception to rape victims in almost all Catholic hospitals in the country.

In addition, the appendices of this report provide a comprehensive overview of Catholic/non-Catholic mergers and affiliations in 1998. They will be a valuable tool for communities facing similar consolidations, as well as for policy makers and hospital administrators. Included are summaries of mergers and affiliations completed, pending, terminated, and suspended in 1998; an updated list of Catholic institutions that are the sole provider of hospital services in their area; and the information gathered from Catholic hospital emergency rooms surveyed to determine the availability of emergency contraception.

During mergers, the Catholic Directives are often extended to non-Catholic facilities-resulting in the curtailment of necessary reproductive health services.

METHODOLOGY

Our tracking of mergers is based primarily on news reports of hospital activities, especially those in *Modern Healthcare*, a prominent trade magazine. Information about the status of reproductive health services was obtained through telephone interviews with hospital administrators or from local and regional advocates. Catholic sole provider hospitals (sole provider in their county) are identified using *Catholic Healthcare in the U.S.A.*, an on-line directory compiled by the Catholic Health Association, and the provider list of the Health Care Financing Administration of the Department of Health and Human Services.

Catholic Health Care Restrictions

Over the last ten years in the United States, hospitals have been consolidating in order to survive in the changing US health care market. These consolidations take many forms. Hospitals can be brought together through a *merger*, which establishes shared assets, liabilities, and administrative functions, or an *acquisition*, the purchase of one facility by another. A lease allows one hospital or health care system to operate another hospital campus for a specified amount of time. Finally, varied *affiliations* and *health networks* may unite hospitals in arrangements such as joint purchasing agreements or sharing of laboratories.

CATHOLIC HEALTH CARE DIRECTIVES

The Catholic health care system, the largest nonprofit effort to deliver health care in the United States, is subject to the same market pressures that drive secular hospitals into consolidations. However, certain aspects of Catholic health care governance make a unique impact on reproductive health services in consolidations in which one partner is Catholic.

While mergers are slowing industry-wide, those involving Catholic hospitals tripled from 1997 to 1998.

Catholic hospitals in the United States are governed by the *Ethical and Religious Directives for Catholic Health Care Services*, issued by the US bishops in 1994.[1] The Directives forbid services that contradict official Catholic teaching. In the area of reproductive health services, the *Directives* specifically prohibit tubal ligations, vasectomies, in vitro fertilization, the prescription or dispensation of contraceptive devices—even condom instruction for patients at risk of contracting HIV/AIDS—and abortions. A hospital that wishes to be "Catholic" is required to have a sponsoring agency approved by the Catholic bishops and must agree to adhere to the Catholic bishops' *Directives*. In addition, links to the pope, local bishop, and sponsoring religious order or diocese allow the church to define the Catholic health care mission and control Catholic health care institutions. These links are maintained through governorship and administration structures, as well as by periodic review—for example, during bishops' periodic visits with the pope, they would be asked to report on the status of some services in their dioceses, including hospitals and other health care institutions.

During negotiations on a merger or affiliation, the Catholic partner will often require the *Directives* to be extended to the non-Catholic facility as a condition of the merger. If the non-Catholic partner complies, patients who need the hospital's reproductive health services lose access to these services.

CREATIVE COMPROMISES

There is no doubt that church regulations complicate mergers. In a merger of a Catholic and non-Catholic hospital, executives must negotiate how the new entity will provide reproductive health services while complying with the dictates of the church hierarchy. But the *Directives* also provide an important and useful tool to reproductive health care advocates. Directive No. 69 specifically allows Catholic hospitals to enter partnerships with non-Catholic facilities that continue to provide a full range of reproductive health services, provided that the Catholic partner limits its involvement with these services:

> *When a Catholic health care institution is participating in a partnership that may be involved in activities judged morally wrong by the Church, the Catholic institution should limit its involvement in accord with the moral principles governing cooperation.*

This Directive makes possible what might be called "creative compromises." Certain hospitals interested in preserving reproductive health services have used this Directive and, as a result, a number of consolidation arrangements allow reproductive health services to continue in a merged facility.

A Year in Review

In the past CFFC has reported on positive trends such as increased community response when services are threatened, new legal tools to block the curtailment of services through mergers, and coalitions that successfully protect reproductive health services in a merging non-Catholic hospital.

What was most striking in 1998 was the continuing explosion of merger activity that began in 1994. Health care industry analysts, including *Modern Healthcare* and Lewin Associates, a consulting firm, had predicted that merger activity would be down in 1998.[2] While mergers are slowing industry-wide, mergers involving Catholic hospitals tripled over the previous year.

EFFECTS ON REPRODUCTIVE HEALTH SERVICES

In 1998, 43 mergers and affiliations between Catholic and non-Catholic hospitals were completed—up from 14 in 1997, 24 in 1996, and 24 in 1995. Of those in 1998, CFFC was able to obtain information on the status of reproductive health services in 36. Eight consolidated entities preserved reproductive health services through creative compromises. For example, in Oakdale, California, and Stamford, Connecticut, public non-Catholic hospitals have continued to provide a wide range of reproductive health services despite an affiliation with or acquisition by a Catholic health system.

However, 17 mergers (47 percent of those on which CFFC was able to obtain information) resulted in the limitation or discontinuation of reproductive health services. In Mid-Island, New York, Catholic Health Services of Long Island and Winthrop South Nassau University Health System spurred community opposition when they attempted an acquisition of Massapequa General that would eliminate reproductive health services in that facility. At the end of 1998, community advocates were attempting to block the state approval required to finalize the acquisition. In a sudden change in consolidation tactics, the health care systems by-passed the state approval process by acquiring Massapequa's property and building, instead of the facility itself, and thereby becoming the hospital's landlord. As a result, the *Directives* have been applied to Massapequa, and reproductive health services have been discontinued.

COMMUNITY RESPONSE

Where communities fought the curtailment of services, they usually succeeded. Community involvement often served as the catalyst for a creative compromise or encouraged hospitals to look for more compatible partners. A community in New York mounted a campaign against the merger of Catholic Benedictine Hospital and non-Catholic Cross River in a

TABLE 1:
Catholic/Non-Catholic Mergers and Affiliations: Impact on Reproductive Health Care

	1990	1991	1992	1993	1994	1995	1996	1997	1998	TOTAL	%
Total	1	0	2	0	19	24	24	14	43	127	—
Total with information available*	1	N/A	2	N/A	14	20	17	10	36	100	100%
All or some reproductive health services discontinued	1	N/A	2	N/A	7	8	9	4	17	48	48%
No significant change in reproductive health services	0	N/A	0	N/A	7	12	8	6	19	52	52%
Nonabortion reproductive health services preserved through creative solutions							4	4	8	16	
Catholic facility merged with non-Catholic facility that did not provide reproductive health services prior to merger							4	2	11	17	

**CFFC was able to obtain information on the status of reproductive health services in 79 percent of the consolidations identified.*

contract that would have curtailed reproductive health services in Cross River's two hospitals, Kingston and Northern Dutchess. After a long and hard fight, assisted by MergerWatch, they persuaded Cross River not to merge if it meant the extension of the *Directives* to its non-Catholic campuses.

BEHIND CLOSED DOORS

Unfortunately, many consolidations that reduced services were finalized with no community input. Only eight of the mergers completed in 1998 had been identified by CFFC at the close of 1997 as pending. The other 35 consolidations were initiated with little public knowledge, and even as negotiations concluded, CFFC and our colleagues were unable to collect information on the status of reproductive health services. Despite the role of hospitals in public health, the merger negotiations were conducted and concluded without much, if any, public scrutiny.

CATHOLIC EVER MORE

Another trend that has continued in 1998 is the purchase of Catholic hospitals by non-Catholic hospital chains. Between 1990 and 1997, CFFC identified ten such acquisitions, and in every case the Catholic hospital, no longer under the governance of the church, continues to abide by the *Directives*. In 1998, another five of these purchases took place, and again, all five hospitals follow the *Directives* and refuse to provide reproductive health services.

CATHOLIC SOLE PROVIDERS

Some Catholic hospitals face no competition because no similar facility is located in the same county, and the number of these "sole providers" continues to grow. These hospitals are communities' only choice for many health services. When a sole provider hospital is Catholic, the area is likely to have little access to reproductive health services. Low-income women, who rely on hospitals for much of their health care and cannot afford to go to a private doctor or travel to distant hospitals, are affected most severely.

In 1997 CFFC identified 76 Catholic sole provider hospitals. In 1998 the number identified has jumped to 91 sole providers, located in 27 states from Vermont to Alaska. Some Catholic sole provider hospitals serve counties where Catholics make up less than one percent of the population. Only five Catholic sole providers are located in counties where the majority of residents are Catholic. In fact, three out of four (68 hospitals) are located in counties where Catholics make up less than 25 percent of the population. Catholic sole provider hospitals enjoy little, if any, competition and, often, higher rates of Medicare reimbursement, while they deny reproductive health care to an entire county.

The reasons for the proliferation of Catholic sole providers remain the same as in 1997. As non-Catholic hospitals in rural areas have closed, Catholic facilities, supported by Catholic health care systems—enlarged by recent mergers and affiliations—have survived. In 1998, an acquisition transformed a non-Catholic sole provider hospital into a Catholic one: the Highland Lakes Medical Center. This sole hospital in Burnet County, Texas, began abiding by the *Directives* after it was acquired by Seton Healthcare Network, a Catholic chain.

CATHOLIC HEALTH ASSOCIATION GETS DEFENSIVE

One goal of tracking Catholic/non-Catholic mergers and affiliations is to raise public awareness. An unintended consequence has been defensiveness among Catholic health care providers. In some cases, administrators of Catholic Health Association member-hospitals refused to answer CFFC's questions over the phone or hung up on researchers, despite the fact that CFFC was requesting public information about the provision of services. In 1998 this defensiveness appeared in the actions of the Catholic Health Association (CHA).

The CHA is the national leadership organization of Catholic health care systems and facilities in the United States. In 1998 CHA joined the ranks of Catholic institutions and individuals who cry "media bias" wherever the news media cover them in a critical way. When *ABC News* joined *National Public Radio*, the *Washington Post*, the *Chicago Tribune*, the *Miami Herald*, *The Nation*, and *USA Today* in covering the rising number of Catholic/non-Catholic consolidations and their effects on reproductive health care, CHA went on the offensive. The impetus was "A Closer Look," a segment on mergers, on ABC's *World News Tonight with Peter Jennings*. After the program aired, Reverend Michael D. Place, president of CHA, wrote a curt letter to David Westin, president of *ABC News*, asserting that the piece contained inaccuracies. Yet the letter offered no proof or alternate data to support CHA's assertion. Coverage of the fact that Catholic hospitals deny reproductive health services may alarm CHA, but it is based on reality, not bias.

So skittish is CHA that it has refused to sell to CFFC publications that are listed on its website as publicly available, and the association denied CFFC access to an audio conference it held on the *Directives*. In addition, CHA has hired Lewin Associates to conduct a review of mergers and acquisitions.[3]

Emergency Contraception: An Emerging Issue

CFFC decided to focus on emergency contraception in this merger update for a number of reasons. First, a concerned nurse practitioner in Houston contacted CFFC about the number of rape victims she sees who have not received the "morning-after pill" in the local Catholic hospital, St. Joseph. She asked us to look into Catholic hospitals' practice patterns for women who have been raped.

Second, the Abortion Access Project of Massachusetts (AAP) undertook an innovative project that inspired us. AAP called the emergency rooms of Catholic hospitals in Massachusetts to ask whether emergency contraception would be offered to rape victims. All but one said no. AAP followed the calls with a letter explaining that the *Directives* allow emergency contraception in Catholic hospitals and emphasizing the importance of offering this to women who have been raped. After receiving this letter, eight Caritas Christi Catholic hospitals scheduled a meeting among themselves to discuss the issue. AAP has not been informed of the results of that meeting.

Third, MergerWatch, which provides hands-on assistance to communities facing mergers, informed CFFC that Catholic hospitals involved in merger negotiations often insist that emergency contraception is not jeopardized by the merger and assert that many Catholic hospitals provide it. But residents of the areas these hospitals serve had indicated to MergerWatch that emergency contraception was not available at the Catholic facilities.

The importance of the issue and the contradictory information in circulation call for an exploration of Catholic positions and hospitals' practices concerning emergency contraception.

THE STANDARD OF CARE

"Emergency contraception" is the use of a drug or device to prevent pregnancy after intercourse.[4] The most widely used form of emergency contraception is a combination of oral contraceptive pills that provide a short, high dose of hormones. Taken within 72 hours of unprotected intercourse, they are 75 percent effective in preventing pregnancy.[5]

Emergency contraception was approved as "remarkably safe and effective" by the Food and Drug Administration on February 25, 1997.[6] Experts at the World Health Organization concluded that emergency contraception has no clinical effect on conditions such as cardiovascular disease, angina, and liver disease.[7] The American College of Obstetricians and Gynecologists states in its 1996 Practice Patterns that "no published studies have reported evidence-based criteria contraindicating use of this [emergency contraception] treatment."[8]

Offering emergency contraception is a medically accepted standard of care for rape victims. Some states require rape victims to be informed of emergency contraception as part of a comprehensive treatment. In fact, in March 1989 a California court ruled that even a Catholic hospital could be held liable for failing to give a rape victim information about and access to emergency contraception. The court concluded that emergency contraception is "pregnancy prevention" and not abortion and so the state "conscience clause," which exempts hospitals from providing abortions, does not apply.[9]

EMERGENCY CONTRACEPTION AFTER RAPE

Catholic positions on emergency contraception are confusing at best: the *Directives* are ambiguous, and Catholic ethicists are in disagreement. Neither CHA, the bishops' conference, nor the Vatican has set definitive rules for the provision of emergency contraception in Catholic hospitals. It is left to the Catholic hospital to interpret the guidance available and determine when to provide emergency contraception.

To the best of our knowledge, no Catholic hospital has a formal family planning program that provides contraceptive pills on a regular basis. Women whose contraception has failed during consensual intercourse receive no emergency contraception in Catholic hospitals.

The *Directives*, however, do treat emergency contraception after rape differently from abortion, sterilization, and contraception for family planning. Directive No. 36 states that "compassionate and understanding care should be given to a person who is the victim of sexual assault. Health care providers should cooperate with law enforcement officials, offer the person psychological and spiritual support, and accurate medical information."

Official teaching in the Catholic church forbids contraception of any type. It only allows periodic abstinence (natural family planning). Rape is distinguished from consensual sex, however, because the sperm is viewed as an extension of the violation, and the woman is seen as having the right to try to prevent further harm by the aggressor, as Pennsylvania's bishops have written.[10]

Another important aspect of Catholic teaching on emergency contraception concerns the process of conception and the definition of abortion. Emergency contraception can prevent pregnancy in a number of ways. It can inhibit ovulation, interfere with the transport of sperm, disrupt fertilization, or prevent implantation in the endometrium.[11] It is this last mode of operation that Catholic hospitals want to avoid. The Catholic church considers anything that interrupts pregnancy after conception to be an abortifacient. The medical field makes implantation the point of distinction, but for the church, once a "new life" has begun, to terminate it is unjust. Therefore, the Catholic church holds that when emergency contraception prevents pregnancy by interfering with implantation, it acts as a method of abortion and is impermissible.[12]

Hospitals may, however, attempt to prevent conception in cases of rape, as Directive No. 36 states:

A female who has been raped should be able to defend herself against a potential conception from the sexual assault. If, after appropriate testing, there is no evidence that conception has occurred already, she may be treated with medications that would prevent ovulation, sperm capacitation or fertilization. It is not permissible, however, to initiate or to recommend treatments that have as their purpose or direct effect the removal, destruction or interference with the implantation of a fertilized ovum.

But the *Directives* do not specify how to determine whether conception has occurred, leaving Catholic hospitals to interpret when they may provide emergency contraception.

ANALYSES FAVORING EMERGENCY CONTRACEPTION

Catholic hospitals provide or refuse to provide emergency contraception for a number of reasons. An overview of five positions follows.

Always Permissible Within 24 Hours: The Process of Conception

One way to deal with the question of whether to provide emergency contraception is by combining Catholic "sanctity of life" considerations with science. The process of conception, which scientists call fertilization, takes approximately one to two days.[13] Before the end of that time, even if a sperm has begun to fertilize an egg, two distinct genetic strands are present. It is not until the end of the process that paternal and maternal genetic materials have merged into a single genetic strand.[14]

Within the church, the understanding that conception is not a moment, but a process, is beginning to take hold. When Archbishop Weakland held a listening session on abortion he came away with this resolution: "I would never be so glib in talking about the 'moment of conception,' since from a medical point of view that is far from accurate: Conception is a long process, not a moment."[15] Under this view, a woman who goes to a Catholic hospital emergency room within 24 hours of being raped should be offered emergency contraception, as there is no possibility that conception has been completed. This practice is entirely consistent with the *Directives*.

Always Permissible: Good Faith

Directive No. 36 (above) calls for "appropriate testing" to determine whether conception has occurred. There is, however, no test that can indicate conclusively whether conception has occurred. It is up to the hospital to decide how to fulfill this requirement while still providing necessary services to rape victims.

Directive No. 36 requires that the hospitals have "no evidence that conception has occurred already"; it does not require confirmation that conception has *not* occurred. Since medical science is not currently able to confirm or deny conception within 72 hours of intercourse, Catholic hospitals are able to provide this service to all women and still follow the *Directives* in good faith.

Always Permissible: Pregnancy Testing

It is fairly routine for many hospitals to administer pregnancy tests prior to emergency contraception to determine if the woman was pregnant prior to being raped. A Catholic hospital might consider a pregnancy test fulfillment of the "appropriate testing" mandate of Directive 36.[16] The administered test *will* come back negative unless the woman was pregnant prior to the rape, and therefore emergency contraception would be administered.

Sometimes Permissible: Ovulation Testing

A much more conservative approach to Directive No. 36 suggests the Catholic hospital should determine whether there is even a *chance* that the woman could conceive. This position recommends not only conducting a pregnancy test, but also questioning the woman about the time of her last menstrual cycle, or even estimating when she ovulated by testing her urine for luteinizing hormone. Reverend Kevin O'Rourke, director of the Center for Health Care Ethics of Saint Louis University and co-author of CHA's *Healthcare Ethics*, is one supporter of this two step approach.

This position may appear reasonable on the surface, but it prevents the use of emergency contraception in almost all cases. Women can only become pregnant if they have intercourse during ovulation or the days just preceding or following ovulation. The purpose of the three tests is to prevent an ovulating woman from receiving emergency contraception. But it is precisely the woman who is ovulating who is at greatest risk of pregnancy after unprotected intercourse. This overly cautious interpretation of the *Directives* only allows emergency contraception to be dispensed to a woman during the times when it is unnecessary.

Never Permissible

The Diocese of Peoria, Illinois, in 1993, and the Archdiocese of Chicago in 1986 went even further than a narrow interpretation of the *Directives* in their position on emergency contraception. The bishops in these dioceses have directed local Catholic hospitals to cease providing emergency contraception even in cases of rape. In Chicago, the Archdiocese even suggested that Catholic hospitals place a warning sticker on the brochures they distribute to rape victims with the message: "Drugs to prevent pregnancy are prescribed at some non-Catholic facilities: Our hospital does not supply these drugs since in good conscience we will not cooperate in what may be an abortion."[17] As a result of this conservatism, in 1992, 14 Catholic hospitals in Chicago denied an estimated 1,004 women access to emergency contraception.[18]

AVAILABILITY OF EMERGENCY CONTRACEPTION

CFFC conducted a nationwide survey of Catholic hospital emergency rooms to determine whether emergency contraception is in fact available to women who request it, regardless of official hospital policy. It is possible that another woman calling the same emergency room would talk with a different staff member and receive a different answer from the one we received. What matters to a woman in crisis, however, is whether the service is accessible to her within the 72-hour window in which emergency contraception is effective.

In our survey, each emergency room was phoned directly by a woman who asked anonymously whether the "morning-after pill," was available. If the answer was a "maybe" or "sometimes," the caller asked for an explanation of the circumstances under which emergency contraception would be provided. If no emergency contraception was available, the caller requested a referral.

Our callers specifically asked for the morning-after pill, the common name given to emergency contraception, and specifically requested a referral. Where the hospital was willing to provide emergency contraception or a referral, we

TABLE 2:
Emergency Contraception Services in Catholic Hospitals
Findings from a nationwide survey of 589 Catholic hospital emergency rooms by Catholics for a Free Choice, Dec. 23, 1998 to Jan. 6, 1999

Provision of Emergency Contraception

	Number	%
Catholic hospital emergency rooms surveyed	589	
Hospital policy is to provide emergency contraception in some cases to women who have been raped	55	9%
Hospital has no policy on emergency contraception	53	9%
Hospital does not provide emergency contraception to women who have been raped	481	82%

Provision of Referral instead of Emergency Contraception

	Number	%
Hospitals denying emergency contraceptives even after rape	481	
Hospital provides referral with phone number, on request	106	22%
Hospital provides referral but no phone number, on request	225	47%
Hospital refuses to provide referral on request	149	31%

do not know whether hospital staff would have offered the medicine or information without first being asked. This is important because many women are unaware of the existence, efficacy, and safety of emergency contraception. For these same reasons, our survey does not determine whether Catholic hospitals are abiding by state laws that require them to inform women who have been raped of the existence of emergency contraception.

We telephoned 589 Catholic hospitals between December 23, 1998 and January 6, 1999. Of those surveyed, 481 (82 percent) said they do not provide women with emergency contraception—even those who have been raped. Where emergency contraception was not available, only 22 percent of emergency rooms provided a useful referral. Of the referrals received, 40 percent were minimal and not terribly helpful—"call the Health Department." In Texas, six hospitals—St. Elizabeth Hospital in Beaumont, Burleson St. Joseph Health Center in Caldwell, St. Paul Medical Center in Dallas, St. Joseph Hospital in Houston, Villa Rosa Hospital in San Antonio, and Providence Health Center in Waco—told the caller that emergency contraception was not available anywhere in the city. In Dillon, South Carolina, Saint Eugene Community Hospital informed the caller that she would have to go to North Carolina to find someone willing to provide emergency contraception.

Eighty two percent of the Catholic hospitals surveyed said they do not provide emergency contraception to women—even those who have been raped.

Fifty-five of the hospitals we called (ten percent) stated that they provided some emergency contraceptive services. Another nine percent of Catholic emergency rooms had no set policies on emergency contraception. Of the 55 emergency rooms that would provide emergency contraception to rape victims, six (11 percent) required that the woman first report the rape to the police.

Sometimes the caller was belittled or chastised. For example, of the 149 emergency rooms that did not provide a referral, staff in 20 hung up on the woman before she could ask for a referral, and those in another 53 were rude. For example, an employee at Bon Secours De Paul Medical Center, Norfolk, Virginia, made no effort to determine the caller's situation before saying, "This is an emergency room, and *that* is not an emergency." The employee then hung up. For a caller who has been raped, "that" certainly feels like an emergency.

Catholic institutions often justify denying emergency contraception by asserting that it is available at non-Catholic facilities and that women who come to Catholic emergency rooms are familiar with the official Catholic position on contraception. But how many women are aware that most Catholic hospitals in the United States refuse emergency contraception even to women who have been raped?

Personnel in some hospitals showed more compassion. In Idaho, one nurse said that, although her hospital would not provide emergency contraception, the caller could take three birth control pills to prevent pregnancy. A woman in a Nebraska hospital offered the home phone number of her own gynecologist, and in Texas, a physician said he would administer the service if the caller could get to the hospital before his shift ended.

Some women are brought to a Catholic hospital by the police because there is no other hospital in the area. In 1998, CFFC identified 91 such Catholic institutions that are the sole provider of hospital services in their areas. Our nationwide survey revealed that 68 of those (75 percent) do not offer emergency contraception, even in cases of rape. The emergency room for sole provider Burleson St. Joseph Regional Health Center in Caldwell, Texas, said that no one in the town offers emergency contraception and provided no referral. In these counties, women who have been raped, as well as women who have had voluntary unprotected sex, have no means of preventing a resulting pregnancy.

Conclusion

It is not only mergers and acquisitions involving Catholic hospitals that limit access to reproductive health services. In all Catholic health care settings, women have little chance of receiving much-needed reproductive health care. As Catholic health care grows and strengthens, the need for research, monitoring, and reporting on this issue grows too.

The case of emergency contraception shows how Catholic health care regulations are on a collision course with new treatment strategies for cases of unprotected sexual activity. And on a question subject to doubt and debate, Catholic hospitals are often favoring abstract theories over women's health needs—even in cases of rape.

Acknowledgements

The extensive research involved in this merger trends update would not have been possible without the assistance of the following Catholics for a Free Choice staff members, who diligently phoned emergency rooms and merger partners to determine the provision of reproductive health services: Megan Hartman, Information Specialist; Rebekah Pinto, Intern; and Amy Scanlon, Communications Assistant.

Notes

[1] Office of Population Research at Princeton University, Emergency Contraception World Wide Web server: http://opr.princeton.edu/ec/

[2] Deanna Bellandi, "Relax, deal pace slowing," *Modern Healthcare*, Jan. 4, 1999.

[3] Randy Hart of Lewin Associates telephoned CFFC on Sept. 15, 1998, asking for clarification on a case in our report *When Catholic and non-Catholic Hospitals Merge: Reproductive Health Compromised.* He confirmed that Lewin was looking at mergers for CHA.

[4] Anna Glasier, "Drug Therapy: Emergency Postcoital Contraception," *New England Journal of Medicine*, Oct. 9, 1997, vol. 337, no. 15.

[5] Office of Population Research at Princeton University, Emergency Contraception World Wide Web server: www.opr.princeton.edu/ec/ecp.html (Jan. 26, 1999).

[6] Food and Drug Administration, "Prescription Productions; Certain Combined Oral Contraceptives for Use as Postcoital Emergency Contraception," *Federal Register*, Feb. 25, 1997, vol. 62, no. 37.

[7] World Health Organization, *Improving Access to Quality Care in Family Planning: Medical Eligibility Criteria for Contraceptive Use* (Geneva: WHO, 1996).

[8] American College of Obstetricians and Gynecologists, *ACOG Practice Patterns: Emergency Oral Contraception* (Washington, DC: ACOG, 1996).

[9] *Brownfield v. Daniel Freeman Marine Hospital*, 208 Cal. App. 3d 405 (1989).

[10] Pennsylvania Catholic Conference, *Guidelines for Catholic Hospitals Treating Victims of Sexual Assault* (Pennsylvania: Pennsylvania Catholic Conference, 1993), as published in Origins, May 4, 1993.

[11] Glasier, op. cit.

[12] While the official Catholic teaching protects life from conception, even conservative moral theologians have argued that it is not until implantation that a unique potential life is created. Before implantation, the zygote or preembryo can still combine or divide; in addition, more than half of fertilizations do not result in live births. Since implantation occurs about seven days after fertilization, emergency contraception within 72 hours cannot be seen as a threat to pregnancy as defined from the moment of implantation.

[13] American College of Obstetricians and Gynecologists, *Preembryo Research: History, Scientific Background, and Ethical Considerations* (Washington, DC: ACOG Committee on Ethics, 1994).

[14] Ibid.

[15] Archbishop Rembert Weakland, "Listening Sessions on Abortion: A Response," *Origins*, May 31, 1990.

[16] Helen Alvaré, a spokesperson for the US National Conference of Catholic Bishops, cited in "Survey Finds Lack of Knowledge Limits Use of Morning-After Pill," *New York Times*, Mar. 29, 1995.

[17] Cecile Bouchardeau, "Catholic Hospitals Deny Rape Victims Choice," *Chicago Reporter*, Oct. 1993.

[18] Ibid.

Appendix A: GLOSSARY

Acquisition: the outright purchase of one facility by another.

Affiliation: a cooperative venture that may entail joint purchasing arrangements, apportionment of medical specialties among separately-owned facilities, or the sharing of laboratory and other ancillary services.

Consolidation: the trend towards mergers and collaborative agreements within the US health care system or, generically, such a contract.

Directives: the *Ethical and Religious Directives for Catholic Health Care Services*, which are promulgated in the United States by the National Conference of Catholic Bishops. Last revised in 1994, the *Directives* outline the mission and spiritual responsibilities of Catholic health care, instruct institutions on maintaining Catholic identity when forming partnerships with non-Catholic health care providers, and prohibit abortion, contraception counseling, in vitro fertilization, fetal tissue research, reproductive sterilization (temporary or permanent), and euthanasia. Where questions arise, the *Directives* are interpreted by the hospital's sponsor and its local bishop.

Emergency Contraception: works to prevent pregnancy after unprotected sexual intercourse. Depending on the time during the menstrual cycle that they are taken, emergency contraceptive pills (ECPs), which can be taken up to 72 hours after unprotected sex, may inhibit or delay ovulation, or they may alter the endometrium (the lining of the uterus), thereby inhibiting implantation of a fertilized egg. The pills are 75 percent effective. The copper-T intrauterine device (IUD) can be inserted up to five days after unprotected intercourse. This latter method reduces the risk of pregnancy by more than 99 percent.[1]

Integrated delivery network, or network: a system that may combine delivery, financing, and management of care in one organization, giving physicians, hospitals, and insurers shared responsibility for health care delivery and risk management.

Lease: a contract under which one health care system or hospital operates another health care facility for a specified time.

Merger: the establishment of shared assets, liabilities, and administrative functions between two entities.

Reproductive health: as defined by the United Nations, "a state of complete physical, mental and social well-being and not merely the absence of disease or infirmity, in all matters relating to the reproductive system and to it functions and processes. Reproductive health therefore implies that people are able to have a satisfying and safe sex life and that they have the capability to reproduce and the freedom to decide if, when and how often to do so."[2]

Reproductive health services: in this report, the reproductive health services discussed are those prohibited by the Directives, as these have been the focus of controversy in mergers between Catholic and non-Catholic hospitals. These services include contraceptive counseling; tubal ligation, vasectomy or other reproductive sterilization, whether temporary or permanent; abortion; emergency contraception for rape victims; and most assisted reproduction services.

Sole provider: sole provider hospitals are hospitals that are the only provider in a given county. Catholic sole provider hospitals were identified using *Catholic Healthcare in the U.S.A.*, an on-line directory complied by the Catholic Health Association and the provider list of the Health Care Financing Administration of the Department of Health and Human Services.

Sponsor: while Catholic hospitals are owned by the church, under canon law, stewardship of each health care facility rests with a sponsoring organization. A sponsor is a Catholic group (religious institute or order, diocese, or private association) which ensures that the hospital follows church guidelines and a specific "healing mission." Sponsors usually have certain governance responsibilities, known as "reserved powers," over their facilities.[3] The sponsor generally appoints and removes the hospital's trustees.

Notes:

[1] Office of Population Research at Princeton University, Emergency Contraception World Wide Web server: www.opr.princeton.edu/ec/ecp.html (Jan. 26, 1999).

[2] United Nations, *Report of the International Conference on Population and Development* (United Nations: Cairo, Oct. 18, 1994), A/CONF.171/13, chapter 7, Sec. 7.2.

[3] *A Profile of the Catholic Healthcare Ministry, 1992* (St. Louis: Catholic Health Association, 1992), p. 82.

Appendix B: 1998 Catholic/Non-Catholic Mergers and Affiliations

CORPORATE

Hospitals: ***Catholic Healthcare West (CHW), San Francisco, CA**
UniHealth, Burbank, CA

Type: Acquisition, December 1998.

Summary: *Reproductive health services limited.* CHW and UniHealth agreed to a merger that gives CHW eight new hospitals. As a result CHW has 14 hospitals in Southern California, including 10 in the Los Angeles area. Now with 46 hospitals statewide, CHW is California's largest hospital operator. UniHealth will continue to support community health efforts as a foundation.

The eight hospitals added to CHW's network reportedly will not become Catholic facilities. However, non-lifesaving abortions and in-vitro fertilizations will not be offered. The parties were expected to close the deal, reportedly worth $300 million, early in 1999.

ARKANSAS

Little Rock

Hospitals: **Columbia Doctors Hospital**
***St. Vincent Health System**

Type: Acquisition, February 1998.

Summary: *Reproductive health services discontinued.* St. Vincent, which also owns St. Vincent's Infirmary Medical Center, purchased 308-bed Columbia Doctors Hospital and renamed it St. Vincent's Doctors Hospital. Before the acquisition, Doctors Hospital performed abortions. The new Doctors Hospital, now a Catholic facility, agreed to follow the Directives and will not provide any reproductive health services.

Little Rock

Hospitals: **Arkansas Women's Health Center**
***St. Vincent's Doctors Hospital (formerly Columbia Doctors Hospital)**

Type: Lease, July 1998.

Summary: *Creative compromise.* Doctors Hospital discontinued reproductive health services in February 1998, when it was purchased by St. Vincent Health System and renamed St. Vincent's Doctors Hospital (see above). In response to this curtailment of services, Arkansas Women's Health Center began leasing space from St. Vincent within Doctors Hospital, near the labor and delivery ward, to perform tubal ligations. Hospital officials have said financial and market pressures forced this joint venture. Arkansas Women's Health Center is reportedly paying for the space by a set amount per sterilization.

This has caused some controversy, including a warning from Pope John Paul II to the local bishop that sterilizations are a sin, according to the *National Catholic Reporter.* The bishop approved the contract but has not commented on the situation.

Rogers

Hospitals: **Rogers Women's Center**
***St. Mary-Rogers Memorial Hospital**

Type: Lease, August 1998.

Summary: *Creative compromise.* St. Mary is negotiating a part-time lease of its obstetrics ward to Rogers Women's Center to perform some reproductive health services. St. Mary is owned by the Sisters of Mercy Health System and staffed by Dominican Sisters. St. Mary officials have told the press that (1) financial and market pressure necessitated the lease and (2) the hospital is following the *Directives*, which allow cooperation and compromise.

*Denotes Catholic entity ✪Denotes public hospital

CALIFORNIA

Los Angeles

Hospitals: ***Queen of Angels-Hollywood Presbyterian Medical Center**
Tenet Healthcare Corp.
Type: Acquisition, May 1998.
Summary: *No lifting of Catholic restrictions after purchase by non-Catholic hospital chain.* California Attorney General Dan Lungren approved the $100 million purchase of 409-bed Queen of Angels by Tenet. The Queen of Angels is engaged in legal battles with the Archdiocese of Los Angeles, which wants final approval of the sale, and with physicians who oppose it.

Oakdale

Hospitals: **✪Oak Valley District Hospital**
***St. Joseph's Regional Health System**
Type: Management agreement, July 1998.
Summary: *Creative compromise.* A 15-year agreement for the management of Oak Valley by St. Joseph's took effect July 1. St. Joseph's is an affiliate of Catholic Healthcare West. Oak Valley staff assured CFFC that they continue to provide reproductive health care, including tubal ligations and contraception.

Redondo Beach

Hospitals: ***Little Company of Mary Health Services**
South Bay Medical Center
Type: Lease, March 1998.
Summary: *Reproductive health services discontinued.* The Beach Cities Health District Board of Trustees voted unanimously to grant a 10-year lease of 149-bed South Bay Medical Center to Little Company of Mary, a Catholic health care system. Little Company strictly abides by the Directives and threatened to pull out of the lease if any restricted services are provided in the leased building. South Bay is considered a Catholic facility for the duration of the lease and abides by the Directives.

San Bernardino

Hospitals: ***Catholic Healthcare West (CHW)**
Community Hospital
Type: Affiliation, August 1998.
Summary: *Reproductive health services limited.* As a member of CHW, 300-bed Community Hospital is now required to follow the Directives, although it will not be a Catholic hospital. The affiliation calls for the elimination of abortions at the hospital and bans in vitro fertilization and artificial insemination, which were not performed at the hospital before the affiliation. According to news reports, tubal ligations, vasectomies, and emergency contraception are allowed, as Community is not a Catholic facility.

Community will be administered by a 15-member board comprising the Community board plus five CHW appointees. This board would vote to decide on any closure or major change in the provision of services at Community; for example, Community could become a Catholic facility if the board approved the change. Community will be jointly managed by another CHW facility, St. Bernardino Medical Center.

There is concern among Community's doctors that the elimination of abortion is the first step toward the prohibition of other family planning services. Local activists had sought a restraining order against the deal but failed to win it.

Taft

Hospitals: ***Catholic Healthcare West (CHW)**
✪West Side District Hospital
Type: Acquisition, August 1998.
Summary: *Reproductive health services discontinued.* CHW acquired 73-bed West Side Hospital and renamed it Mercy West Side Hospital. The hospital is administered by CHW but not considered a Catholic facility, according to West Side, but it does abide by the Directives. Mercy West Side has no obstetrician/gynecologists on staff.

CONNECTICUT

Stamford

Hospitals: ***St. Joseph Medical Center**
✪Stamford Health System
Type: Acquisition, November 1998.
Summary: *Creative compromise.* In a process that began in December 1996, Stamford Health System has acquired 51 percent of St. Joseph Medical Center from St. Vincent's Health Services, a Catholic system, for $6 million. Stamford remains a community hospital and provides a wide range of reproductive health services, including contraception and abortion.

St. Joseph's is set to be demolished and rebuilt by 2002. The acquisition contract states, however, that no reproductive health services can ever be offered at the St. Joseph siteÑeven in a rebuilt and renamed facility. This deal, essentially a creative compromise, preserved reproductive health services because Stamford purchased St. Joseph.

Westport
Hospitals: **Hall-Brooke Hospital**
***St. Vincent's Health Services**
Type: Acquisition, November 1998.
Summary: *Reproductive health services were not offered prior to acquisition.* St. Vincent's, which owns St. Vincent's Medical Center, acquired 70-bed Hall-Brooke Hospital, a psychiatric hospital in Westport. Under the agreement, Hall-Brooke becomes a Catholic hospital abiding by the *Directives.*

ILLINOIS

Chicago
Hospitals: ***Resurrection Health Care**
Westlake Community Hospital
Westlake Health System
Type: Acquisition, July 1998.
Summary: *Reproductive health services discontinued.* Resurrection, a four-hospital Catholic system, acquired Westlake Health System, the owner of 239-bed Westlake Community Hospital. Westlake administrators said they have agreed to follow the *Directives* as a condition of the merger.

INDIANA

Fort Wayne
Hospitals: **Quorum**
***St. Joseph Medical Center**
Type: Acquisition, July 1998.
Summary: *No lifting of Catholic restrictions after purchase by non-Catholic system.* Quorum has acquired 175-bed St. Joseph Medical Center from Ancilla Systems, a Catholic chain. St. Joseph will continue to abide by the *Directives*, although Quorum remains a non-Catholic health system.

Indianapolis
Hospitals: **Health Services of Indianapolis**
Lifelines Children's Hospital
*St. Vincent Hospital
Type: Acquisition, September 1998.
Summary: *Reproductive health services were not offered prior to acquisition.* In early 1998, St. Vincent Hospital and Health Services of Indianapolis signed an agreement to purchase Lifelines Children's Hospital. The Daughters of Charity National Health System, which owns St. Vincent, has since approved the agreement. Lifelines Children's Hospital did not offer reproductive health services prior to the acquisition, but CFFC's request for information regarding the Directives and Lifelines was denied.

Lafayette
Hospitals: **Lafayette Home Hospital**
***St. Elizabeth Medical Center**
Type: Merger, September 1998.
Summary: *CFFC's request for information denied.* A review of this merger by the US Department of Justice ended with no action. The 205-bed St. Elizabeth has merged with 280-bed Lafayette to form Greater Lafayette Health Services, which follows the *Directives.* The local bishop has approved but not announced an agreement concerning reproductive health services.

KANSAS

Kansas City
Hospitals: **Bethany Medical Center**
***Sisters of Charity of Leavenworth Health Services Corp.**
Type: Acquisition, December 1998.
Summary: *Reproductive health services discontinued.* The Sisters of Charity acquired 240-bed Bethany Medical Center from Columbia. All reproductive health services, including tubal ligations and contraception, have been discontinued at Bethany, which is now considered a Catholic facility and abides by the *Directives.*

*Denotes Catholic entity ✪Denotes public hospital

KENTUCKY

Lexington

Hospitals: ***Catholic Health Initiatives (CHI)**
Jewish Hospital Lexington

Type: Acquisition, December 1998.

Summary: *Reproductive health services discontinued.* Jewish Hospital HealthCare Services sold the 174-bed Jewish Hospital Lexington to CHI. The facility was renamed St. Joseph's East and abides by the *Directives.*

LOUISIANA

Coushatta

Hospitals: **L.S. Huchabat M.D. Memorial Hospital**
***Sisters of Charity Health Care System**

Type: Acquisition, 1998.

Summary: *CFFC's request for information denied.* The Houston-based Sisters of Charity Health Care System bought 74-bed Huchabat.

MARYLAND

Towson

Hospitals: ***St. Joseph Medical Center**
Upper Chesapeake Health System

Type: Partnership, January 1998.

Summary: *Creative compromise.* Upper Chesapeake Health System is not required to follow the *Directives* and does not follow them.

MICHIGAN

Farmington Hills

Hospitals: ***Mercy Health Services**
Muskegon General Hospital

Type: Merger, November 1998.

Summary: *Reproductive health services discontinued.* Mercy Health Services acquired 127-bed Muskegon General Hospital for $7.5 million, merging its own 175-bed Mercy Hospital together with Muskegon as Mercy General Health Partners. The merger, which follows a three-year joint operation agreement between the two hospitals, consolidated clinical operations and converted Muskegon's emergency room into an urgent-care center. The facility that was Muskegon now abides by the *Directives* and has discontinued all reproductive health services.

Kalamazoo

Hospitals: ***Borgess Health Alliance**
Doctors Hospital

Type: Merger, March 1998.

Summary: *Reproductive health services were not offered prior to merger.* The merger of Borgess and the 46-bed Doctors created a four-hospital Catholic system. Doctors Hospital, which did not offer reproductive health services before the merger, became a Catholic facility and follows the *Directives.*

Pontiac

Hospitals: **Pontiac Osteopathic Hospital Medical Center (POH)**
***St. John Health System**

Type: Affiliation, October 1998.

Summary: *CFFC's request for information denied.* St. John's, which is owned by the Sisters of St. Joseph, and POH signed an agreement under which they will collaborate on graduate medical education programs for osteopathic medicine, managed-care contracting, and group purchasing but retain ownership and control of their own facilities. St. John will also allow POH access to its mobile magnetic resonance imaging unit. A POH spokesperson declined to say which reproductive health services it currently offers.

MINNESOTA

Farmington

Hospitals: ***Benedictine Health System**
South Suburban Medical Center

Type: Acquisition, January 1998.

Summary: *Reproductive health services discontinued.* Benedictine acquired the 95-bed South Suburban Medical Center. The acquired hospital, called Trinity, is Catholic and has discontinued all reproductive health services.

Long Prairie

Hospitals: ***CentraCare**
Long Prairie Memorial Hospital and Home

Type: Acquisition, January 1998.

Summary: *CFFC's request for information denied.* CentraCare, the Catholic parent of 616-bed St. Cloud Hospital, purchased 141-bed Long Prairie Memorial for $3.2 million.

MISSOURI

St. Louis

Hospitals: ***St. Louis University Hospital**
Tenet Healthcare Corp.

Type: Acquisition, March 1998.

Summary: *No lifting of Catholic restrictions after purchase by non-Catholic hospital chain.* Tenet acquired 303-bed St. Louis University Hospital for $300 million. Despite its non-Catholic ownership, St. Louis University Hospital continues to abide by the *Directives*, as a condition of the transfer of ownership.

NEW JERSEY

Willingboro

Hospitals: **Allegheny University Hospital-Rancocas**
***Our Lady of Lourdes Medical Center**

Type: Acquisition, December 1998.

Summary: *Reproductive health services discontinued.* Our Lady of Lourdes, part of Catholic Health East, purchased Allegheny University Hospital-Rancocas for an undisclosed sum. Allegheny is becoming a Catholic hospital that will abide by the *Directives* and will not provide any reproductive health services. At the time of acquisition, abortions immediately ceased. Other services are being phased out.

NEW YORK

Long Island

Hospitals: ***Catholic Health Services of Long Island**
Massapequa General Hospital
Winthrop South Nassau University Health System

Type: Lease, December 1998.

Summary: *Reproductive health services discontinued.* Catholic Health Services of Long Island had been working toward purchasing Massapequa General Hospital but then, instead, teamed up with Winthrop South Nassau University Health System to buy Massapequa's real estate. Massapequa General has become their tenant. Local advocates for continuing reproductive health services at Massapequa were surprised to discover that this change of strategy immediately transformed the power shift from an acquisition, which would have required state approval, into a lease, which does not. As a result the *Directives* have been extended to Massapequa, and all reproductive health care services have been eliminated.

West Haverstraw

Hospitals: ***Catholic Healthcare Network**
✪Helen Hayes Hospital

Type: Affiliation, August 1998.

Summary: *Reproductive health services were not offered prior to affiliation.* Helen Hayes, a 155-bed state-run public hospital, joined the 37-member Catholic Healthcare Network as an affiliate, becoming only the second non-Catholic facility to do so. Like All Catholic Healthcare Network members, Helen Hayes has agreed to follow the *Directives.* Helen Hayes is a physical rehabilitation hospital with no emergency services and offered no reproductive health services before the affiliation.

NORTH CAROLINA

Asheville

Hospitals: **Memorial Mission Medical Center**
***Sisters of Mercy of North Carolina**
***St. Joseph's Hospital**

Type: Acquisition, November 1998.

Summary: *No lifting of Catholic restrictions after purchase by non-Catholic medical center.* Sisters of Mercy is selling 264-bed St. Joseph's Hospital to Memorial Mission Medical Center for $90 million. This deal between Asheville's only private, acute-care hospitals follows their earlier "virtual merger" through contracting arrangements (which had required an expansion of the state's antitrust exemption law). St. Joseph's, the last remaining Catholic hospital in the state, continues to follow the *Directives* despite its ownership by a non-Catholic health care system.

NORTH DAKOTA

Minot

Hospitals: **Quorum**
***Sisters of St. Francis of Denver**
UniMed Medical Center

Type: Acquisition, March 1998.

Summary: *No lifting of Catholic restrictions after purchase by non-Catholic health system.* Quorum acquired UniMed Medical Center from the Sisters of St. Francis of Denver. UniMed includes St. Joseph's Hospital, a Catholic institution that continues to abide by the *Directives* despite its ownership by a for-profit system.

*Denotes Catholic entity ✪Denotes public hospital

OKLAHOMA

Enid

Hospitals: **Integris Bass Baptist Health Center**
***St. Mary's Mercy Hospital**

Type: Joint Venture, 1998.

Summary: *Reproductive health services to be discontinued.* St. Mary's and Integris Bass plan to build a $14 million medical center, to be called the Plaza for Women and Infants, which will become the region's lone birthing facility. Although Integris now offers tubal ligations, but it will discontinue them and the new facility will operate strictly by the *Directives*. The Plaza will not provide tubal ligations, nor will its health education program offer contraceptive information. Doctors have not even been able to learn whether they will be allowed to provide contraceptive counseling and devices in their new offices at the Plaza.

A community coalition is challenging the curtailment of services. Prochoice state legislator Rep. Laura Boyd, who opposes the abridgement of reproductive health services, has hosted three community meetings to discuss the joint venture, and residents formed a group called Oklahoma Coalition for Quality in Women's Health Care to protect access to reproductive health services.

OREGON

Cottage Grove

Hospitals: **Cottage Grove Hospital**
***PeaceHealth Health Services**

Type: Affiliation, August 1998. Acquisition of assets pending.

Summary: *CFFC's request for information denied.* Cottage Grove signed an agreement with PeaceHealth for a $1.5 million line of credit and hired PeaceHealth to Cottage Grove Clinic, as Cottage Grove Hospital was closing for financial reasons. Since then, Southland Medical Groups of PeaceHealth has been operating Cottage Grove Clinic, which has no in-patient facilities. A court is to meet in February to consider PeaceHealth's bid to acquire the assets of Cottage Grove. PeaceHealth has not decided whether to reopen Cottage Grove, if the acquisition is approved, nor whether reproductive health services would resume there, a PeaceHealth spokesperson said.

PENNSYLVANIA

Philadelphia

Hospitals: ***Mercy Health System**
St. Ignatius Nursing Home of West Philadelphia

Type: Affiliation, October 1998.

Summary: *Reproductive health services were not offered prior to affiliation.* Mercy and St. Ignatius do not plan to merge their assets.

Philadelphia

Hospitals: ***Catholic Health Initiatives (CHI)**
University of Pennsylvania Health System (UPHS)

Type: Affiliation, September 1998.

Summary: *Creative compromise.* The 11 UPHS hospitals and CHI's five Philadelphia-area hospitals reached a 10-year contract. The affiliation, which is expected to include cooperative managed care contracting, will broaden the geographic reach of UPHS tertiary clinical services and enhance primary-care delivery in the metropolitan area. UPHS plans to share its expertise in health and disease management with the hospitals CHI's nationwide network. The *Directives* have not been extended to the UPHS facilities, but any joint initiatives of the two systems would abide by the *Directives*.

SOUTH CAROLINA

Charleston

Hospitals: ***Bon Secours Health System**
Carolinas HealthCare System
Medical Society of South Carolina

Type: Partnership, July 1998.

Summary: *Reproductive health services limited.* The not-for-profit Medical Society of South Carolina, Bon Secours Health System of Marriottsville, MD, and Carolinas HealthCare System of Charlotte, NC, agreed to a mergerlike partnership under a new company, Care Alliance Health Services. The medical society owns Roper CareAlliance, the 380-bed Roper Hospital, and the 104-bed Roper Hospital North. Bon Secours owns 165-bed Bon Secours-St. Francis Xavier Hospital. A supermajority of the 13-member board of CareAlliance Health Services must be local residents, and each facility will have its own local advisory board.

According to a Roper spokesperson, Bon Secours-St. Francis Xavier exercises no control over Roper's provision of services. In September 1997, however, a Roper spokesperson told CFFC abortions would be barred as a condition of the merger.

Dillon

Hospitals: **McLeod Regional Medical Center**
***Saint Eugene Medical Center**

Type: Acquisition, January 1998.

Summary: *Reproductive health services were not offered prior to acquisition.* The 421-bed McLeod, a Christian facility, acquired 92-bed Saint Eugene from St. Louis-based SSM Health Care System. No reproductive health services were provided at McLeod before it acquired Saint Eugene.

TEXAS

Austin

Hospitals: **Central Texas Medical Foundation (CTMF)**
***Seton Healthcare Network**

Type: Acquisition, March 1998.

Summary: *CFFC's request for information denied.* Seton purchased CTMF for $1.1 million. CTMF trains residents at seven outpatient clinics, some of which provide a wide range of reproductive health services that can include abortions. CFFC's request for information on how the *Directives* will effect CTMF was denied.

Austin

Hospitals: ***Seton Healthcare Network**
Shoal Creek Hospital

Type: Acquisition, May 1998.

Summary: *Reproductive health services discontinued.* Seton bought 151-bed Shoal Creek Hospital, renaming it Seton Shoal Creek Hospital. Now a Catholic hospital abiding by the *Directives*, Shoal Creek no longer provides reproductive health services.

Burnet

Hospitals: **✪Highland Lakes Medical Center**
***Seton Healthcare Network**

Type: Acquisition, February 1998.

Summary: *Reproductive health services discontinued.* Seton bought 42-bed Highland Lakes and renamed the Burnet, Texas, hospital Seton Highland Lakes. Once acquired, Highland Lakes became a Catholic facility, abiding by the *Directives*, and eliminated all reproductive health services.

Lubbock

Hospitals: **Lubbock Methodist Hospital System**
***St. Mary of the Plains Hospital**

Type: Merger, June 1998.

Summary: *Reproductive health services limited.* After more than two years of negotiation, 415-bed St. Mary of the Plains and 644-bed Lubbock Methodist merged to form Covenant Health System, valued at $600 million. The Federal Trade Commission cleared the merger last year and Methodist agreed to pay an undisclosed sum to settle a dispute with the Internal Revenue Service over its tax-exempt status. Both campuses abide by the *Directives*. According to the Human Services Department of Lubbock, Covenant provides a space for performing tubal ligations but does not accept any proceeds from the provision of this service.

WEST VIRGINIA

Huntington

Hospitals: **Cabell Huntington**
Pleasant Valley Hospital
***Saint Mary's Hospital**

Type: Affiliation, January 1998.

Summary: *Creative compromise.* A mergerlike arrangement united 293-bed Cabell, 201-bed Pleasant Valley, and 440-bed Saint Mary's into a partnership called Genesis. The *Directives* do not apply to the Cabell Huntington and Pleasant Valley campuses.

*Denotes Catholic entity ✪Denotes public hospital

WISCONSIN

Kenosha

Hospitals: **Kenosha Hospital and Medical Center**
***St. Catherine's Hospital**

Type: Holding company created, 1998.

Summary: *CFFC's request for information denied.* Without merging assets, 148-bed St. Catherine's and 116-bed Kenosha created a holding company to oversee the hospitals' operations.

Fox Valley

Hospitals: ***Ministry Health Care**
Network Health System

Type: Affiliation, October 1998.

Summary: *Creative compromise.* The affiliation between Ministry Health Care and Network Health System maintains the corporations' individuality where reproductive health services are concerned. None of the Catholic and non-Catholic hospitals Ministry owns will change any of the services they provide. Network Health System is comprised of La Salle Clinic, a family practice, and Network Health Plan of Wisconsin. Network Health Plan will not follow the *Directives* and will continue to provide contraceptive services under some health plans. La Salle will continue providing contraceptive services and tubal ligations.

Ministry Health Care includes Saint Joseph's Hospital in Marshfield, Saint Michael's Hospital in Stevens Point, Sacred Heart Hospital in Tomahawk, and Saint Mary's Hospital in Rhinelander—all of them Catholic—as well as the non-Catholic Rhinelander Regional Medical Group and its affiliated Eagle River, Tomahawk, and Crandon hospitals.

Appendix C: Recently Terminated or Suspended Consolidation Negotiations

FLORIDA

South Miami

Hospitals: **Baptist Hospital**
***Mercy Hospital**

Outcome: Merger negotiations terminated, July 1998.

Summary: In 1997, Baptist adopted a policy banning abortions but denied the policy was part of a deal being negotiated with Mercy. A local coalition assisted by CFFC and MergerWatch exposed the potential impact on reproductive health services of a merger between Mercy and Baptist. In 1998, Baptist's board of trustees announced it would change its abortion policy to allow abortions in one of Baptist's facilities, South Miami Hospital. Mercy then scrapped the merger, having announced earlier that it would not merge with a facility that provides abortions.

ILLINOIS

Rockford

Hospitals: ***Saint Anthony Medical Center**
SwedishAmerican Hospital

Outcome: Merger negotiations terminated, June 1998.

Summary: After 14 months of negotiation and antitrust clearance from the US Department of Justice, SwedishAmerican withdrew from the proposed merger. The hospitals declined to provide a reason for abruptly ending talks.

INDIANA

Indianapolis and Beech Grove

Hospitals: **Community Hospitals**
***St. Francis Hospital and Health Centers**

Outcome: Joint venture negotiations terminated, January 1999.

Summary: Community Hospitals, a four-hospital system, had signed an agreement with two-hospital St. Francis to form a joint operating company. A board of directors was to have governed the company with equal representation from both systems. The deal fell through for undisclosed reasons.

MARYLAND

Baltimore

Hospitals: **Greater Baltimore Medical Center (GBMC)**
***St. Joseph's Medical Center**

Outcome: Merger negotiations terminated, June 1998.

Summary: After months of debate over how the *Directives* would affect the provision of reproductive health services at GBMC, including a proposed ban on abortions, the GBMC trustees fell one vote short of the two-thirds majority needed to approve the partnership with St. Joseph's. The potential loss of reproductive health services at GBMC, which includes the Hospital for the Women of Maryland, had concerned members of the GBMC endowment fund. According to MergerWatch, the board of the Hospital for Women planned to withdraw financial support from GBMC if the merger occurred.

Baltimore

Hospitals: ***Mercy Medical Center**
North Arundel Hospital

Outcome: Merger negotiations terminated, May 1998.

Summary: A spokesperson for Mercy Medical Center would not elaborate on why the merger plans were terminated.

MASSACHUSETTS

Holyoke

Hospitals: **Holyoke Hospital**
***Providence Hospital**

Outcome: Merger negotiations terminated, June 1998.

Summary: Holyoke Hospital backed out of the deal because of concerns that a merger would result in the "loss of services" at the non-Catholic campus by making the nearby Catholic hospital the dominant service provider, a spokesperson for Holyoke Hospital said.

*Denotes Catholic entity ✪Denotes public hospital

MISSOURI

Cape Girardeau

Hospitals: ***Saint Francis Medical Center**
Southeast Missouri Hospital

Outcome: Merger negotiations terminated, January 1998.

Summary: The 264-bed Saint Francis and 243-bed Southeast had said that if they failed to merge, one hospital or the other would be bought by a national health system. They hoped to complete their merger without community opposition, but area residents complained to the justice department about the planned curtailment of reproductive health services. The attorney general blocked the merger for antitrust reasons.

NEW YORK

Hospitals: **Mid-Hudson Valley**
***Benedictine Hospital**
Cross River Inc. (Kingston and Northern Dutchess hospitals)

Outcome: Merger negotiations terminated, July 1998.

Summary: The *Directives* had been expected to apply to this three-hospital merger. The first phase of the deal was completed in early 1998, when the two non-Catholic hospitals united to form Cross River Healthcare. The next phase was to have been the merger of Cross River with Benedictine. In the face of community opposition, however, Kingston and Northern Dutchess abruptly dissolved their own merger and terminated negotiations with the Catholic hospital.

The controversy over the negotiations reached into nearby New York Medical College, a Catholic school. Because the merger was expected to eliminate access to reproductive health services, Dr. David Mesches, chairman of family medicine at the college, agreed to lease space in his medical offices for the provision of abortions. Dr. Mesches was removed from his position as chairman after he was quoted in the press on the legality of abortion. He later resigned his faculty position as well.

Niagara Falls

Hospitals: ***Mount St. Mary's Medical Center**
Niagara Falls Memorial Medical Center

Outcome: Merger negotiations temporarily terminated.

Summary: Niagara and Mount St. Mary's (a Daughters of Charity hospital) have called off their merger negotiations, but community activists involved in blocking the merger are not certain that reproductive health services are safe at Niagara Falls Memorial. The two hospitals remain in affiliation with each other, as Health System of Niagara, which was to have been a step toward full merger. If the merger is ever completed, Niagara would be required to abide by the *Directives* and eliminate reproductive health services.

PENNSYLVANIA

Erie

Hospitals: **Hamot Medical Center**
***Saint Vincent Health Center**

Outcome: Merger negotiations terminated, August 1998.

Summary: Hamot and Saint Vincent called off the merger they had been negotiating since November 1996. The deal was derailed by the conditions that Pennsylvania's attorney general stipulated for its approval. Hamot's chief executive said the conditions were "challenging" but "not unreasonable or undoable," but Saint Vincent found them unacceptable.

Lancaster

Hospitals: **Community Hospital**
***St. Joseph Hospital**

Outcome: Joint operating agreement negotiations terminated, 1998.

Summary: In August 1998, 256-bed St. Joseph Hospital and 142-bed Community Hospital signed a letter of interest to explore a joint operating agreement. But negotiations quickly terminated, and a for-profit group bought Community Hospital.

Philadelphia

Hospitals: **Jefferson Health System**
***Mercy Health Corp. of Southeastern Pennsylvania**

Outcome: Alliance negotiations terminated, 1998.

Summary: Tentative agreement had been reached on an alliance in which Mercy and Jefferson would undertake joint initiatives while maintaining separate ownership and historic assets. The alliance was called off, however.

TENNESSEE

Nashville

Hospitals: **Baptist Hospital**
***Saint Thomas Health Services**

Outcome: Merger negotiations suspended, May 1998.

Summary: Merger talks were suspended. Hospital administrators declined to say why but confirmed that they expect discussions to begin again soon.

Appendix D: Pending Consolidations

MULTISTATE

California—San Jose
Illinois—*Hoffman Estates

Hospitals: **Alexian Brothers Hospital**
Columbia

Type: Acquisition pending.

Summary: Alexian Brothers Health System, based in Illinois, and Columbia scheduled a swap of Alexian Brothers Hospital in San Jose and two of its affiliates in California for two of Columbia's hospitals in Illinois. After protests from San Jose Bishop R. Pierre DuMaine as well as San Jose residents and public officials, the swap was postponed. Bishop DuMaine said he opposed the swap because negotiations had not included anyone from the Catholic or health care communities in San Jose.

ILLINOIS

Morris

Hospitals: **Morris Hospital**
***St. Joseph Medical Center/Franciscan Sisters Health Care Corp.**

Type: Affiliation pending.

Summary: A Morris Hospital administrator says negotiations to affiliate are proceeding. During negotiations, Morris continues to operate under its own regulations, and reproductive health services are available.

INDIANA

Evansville

Hospitals: ***St. Mary's Medical Center**
Welborn Memorial Baptist Hospital

Type: Acquisition pending.

Summary: *Directives expected to apply.* The 488-bed St. Mary's, an affiliate of Daughters of Charity National Health System, is to acquire 274-bed Welborn Memorial Baptist Hospital. The hospitals signed a letter of intent in March 1998, and received federal antitrust clearance in the fall. Welborn Hospital will terminate all reproductive health services after it is acquired, including provision of contraceptive counseling and devices, tubal ligations, and in vitro fertilization, a hospital spokesperson said.

MICHIGAN

Kalamazoo

Hospitals: ***Borgess Health Alliance**
Metropolitan Health Corp.

Type: Joint operation pending.

Summary: Metropolitan Health and Borgess signed a letter of intent to form a 50-50 joint operating company, expected to come together by mid-1999. Metropolitan Health is the parent of 250-bed Metropolitan Hospital, which is expected to continue providing reproductive health services and not to abide by the *Directives.*

Mount Clemens

Hospitals: **Mount Clemens General Hospital**
***St. Joseph's Mercy of Macomb**

Type: Affiliation pending.

Summary: Mount Clemens had been considering affiliation proposals from four health systems in Michigan: St. John Health System, a Catholic system in Detroit; Detroit Medical Center; William Beaumont Hospital, Royal Oak; and its neighbor St. Joseph's. Mount Clemens and St. Joseph's, Macomb County's two largest health systems, recently entered a "period of exclusive discussion" with each other, which they expect to complete early in 1999. A Mount Clemens spokesperson said it is too early to tell whether Mount Clemens would adhere to the *Directives.*

NEW JERSEY

Roseland

Hospitals: **Elizabeth General Medical Center**
***St. Elizabeth Hospital**

Type: Merger pending.

Summary: *Directives expected to apply.* St. Elizabeth Hospital signed a definitive merger agreement with the

*Denotes Catholic entity ✪Denotes public hospital

445-bed Elizabeth General Medical Center and expects to close the deal by the end of March 1999. The proposed merger would create a parent organization, under which Elizabeth General would become a Catholic institution and abide by the Directives. According to a spokesperson for Elizabeth General, reproductive health services including tubal ligations would be prohibited after the merger.

NEW YORK

Batavia

Hospitals: Genesee Memorial Hospital
*St. Jerome Hospital

Type: Merger pending.

Summary: *Directives expected to apply.* The 70-bed Genesee and the 96-bed St. Jerome have proposed the creation of a new company owned 50-50 by the private not-for-profit group that runs Genesee and St. Jerome's sponsoring company, Catholic Health System of Western New York. Once the merger is complete, the Genesee campus will be required to follow the *Directives*, and all reproductive health services will be eliminated.

Gloversville

Hospitals: Nathan Littauer Hospital and Nursing Home
*St. Mary's Hospital

Type: Affiliation pending.

Summary: *Directives expected to apply.* The boards of Littauer and St. Mary's approved an agreement to create a new parent company to oversee both hospitals. Each hospital will have equal representation on the governing board. Littauer has reportedly agreed to stop performing abortions (about 50 are performed there each year now) but will continue other reproductive health services, including tubal ligations. Littauer and St. Mary's, part of St. Louis-based Carondelet Health System, are expected to close their deal in the spring of 1999, although they still need approvals from the bishop of Albany and state hospital regulators.

Long Island

Hospitals: *Catholic Health Services of Long Island
Mid-Island Hospital
Winthrop South Nassau University Health System

Type: Acquisition pending.

Summary: *Directives expected to apply.* The acquisition of Mid-Island by Catholic Health Services and Winthrop South Nassau is awaiting state approval. After the acquisition Mid-Island will follow the *Directives* and stop reproductive health services, including abortions and sterilizations—both of which it frequently provides.

PENNSYLVANIA

Johntown

Hospital: *Bon Secours-Holy Family Regional Health System
Conemaugh Health System

Type: Affiliation pending.

Summary: *Directives expected to apply.* Bon Secours and Conemaugh are negotiating a link and at the end of 1998 were conducting due diligence. Conemaugh expects to follow the *Directives* after the deal is finalized.

TEXAS

Beaumont

Hospital: Beaumont Medical and Surgical Hospital
Silsbee Doctors Hospital
*Sisters of Charity

Type: Acquisition pending.

Summary: *Directives expected to apply.* The Sisters of Charity have signed a letter of intent to buy 59-bed Silsbee and 364-bed Beaumont Medical. Sisters of Charity, which also owns Beaumont's only other hospital, St. Elizabeth, does not offer contraceptive services and allows sterilizations only on a doctor's recommendation. The local chapter of the National Organization for Women launched a letter writing campaign to urge government officials to block the purchase because it would require women to travel to Galveston for tubal ligations. Opposition is also coming from community members opposed to the prospect that St. Elizabeth and the Sisters of Charity, which already control 60 percent of the market for hospital services in Beaumont, would gain an additional 20-25 percent share.

Dallas

Hospital: ✪Parkland Hospital
*St. Paul Medical Center

Type: Lease pending.

Summary: Parkland Hospital, a 940-bed facility, is discussing the possible lease of St. Paul, a facility licensed for 540-beds but currently staffing only 308-beds. If the lease is signed, as is expected in the spring of 1999, St. Paul would retain its name and Catholic affiliation.

Luling

Hospital: **Edgar B. Davis Memorial Hospital**
***Seton Healthcare Network**

Type: Lease pending.

Summary: Seton is negotiating a 30-year lease, expected to be signed in February 1999, to gain control of 30-bed Edgar B. Davis, which is expected to close on February 1. A Davis spokesperson said it is unclear whether the leased hospital will abide by the *Directives*.

VIRGINIA

Newport News and Gloucester

Hospital: ***Mary Immaculate Hospital**
Riverside Health System

Type: Affiliation pending.

Summary: Riverside and Mary Immaculate both voted in August to pursue an affiliation, which is expected to be finalized in February 1999. The two hospitals would be run by a joint operating company but would retain separate boards and staffs. The provision of reproductive health services is one of the issues the two hospitals plan to resolve before finalizing the affiliation. Riverside performs many tubal ligations, some vasectomies, and few abortions. Compromises being considered include using separately funded operating rooms or moving all reproductive health services to a separate facility not included in the alliance. At this time Riverside hopes to continue all reproductive health services.

*Denotes Catholic entity ✪Denotes public hospital

Appendix E: Mergers and Affiliations Within Catholic Health Care, 1998

COMPLETED:

MULTISTATE

*St. John's Health System, Tulsa, OK
*Via Caritas Health System, Denville, NJ
*Via Christi Health System, Wichita, KS
*Via Christi Health System, Wisconsin Branch
*Allegany Health Systems, Tampa, FL
*Eastern Mercy Health System, Radnor, PA
*Sisters of Providence Health System, Springfield, MI

BY STATE:

CALIFORNIA

Los Angeles
*Catholic Healthcare West's Southern California division
*Little Company of Mary Health Services

INDIANA

Kokomo
*Saint Joseph Hospital and Health Center
*St. Vincent Hospitals and Health Services

NEW YORK

Staten Island
*Bayley Seton Hospital
*St. Vincent's Medical Center of Richmond

*Denotes Catholic entity ✪Denotes public hospital

PENDING:

MULTISTATE

*Catholic Healthcare Partners, Cincinnati, OH
*Franciscan Health Partnership, Albany, NY
*Daughters of Charity National Health System, St. Louis, MO
*Sisters of St. Joseph Health System, Ann Arbor, MI
*Incarnate Word Health System, San Antonio, TX
*Sisters of Charity Health Care System, Houston, TX

BY STATE:

GEORGIA

Athens
*Congregation of the Missionary Sisters of the Sacred Heart of Jesus
*Sisters of Mercy of the Americas
*St. Mary's Hospital

INDIANA

Crown Point
*Sisters of St. Francis Health Services
*St. Anthony Medical Center

MICHIGAN

Livonia
*Sisters of Mercy, Detroit Regional Community—Mercy Health Services, Farmington Hills
*Felician Sisters of Livonia—St. Mary Hospital of Livonia

NEW YORK

New York
*Catholic Medical Center of Brooklyn and Queens
*Saint Vincents Hospital and Medical Center of New York
*Sisters of Charity Healthcare System

RHODE ISLAND

Providence
*Caritas Christi Health Care System
*St. Joseph Health Services

Appendix F: Catholic Sole Provider Hospitals

In 1998, the Health Care Financing Administration of the US Department of Health and Human Services listed 1604 hospitals that are the "sole providers" of hospital services in their counties. Currently, 91 Catholic hospitals, in 27 states from Vermont to Alaska, are designated sole providers.

Only five Catholic sole providers are located in counties where most residents are Catholic. In fact, three-fourths (68 hospitals) are in counties where Catholics make up less than 25 percent of the population.

Hospital	Location	County Population	% Catholic
ALASKA			
Ketchikan General Hospital	Ketchikan Ketchikan County	13,828	8.7%
Providence Kodiak Island Medical Center	Kodiak Kodiak Island County	13,309	4.5%
ARIZONA			
Carondelet Holy Cross Hospital	Nogales Santa Cruz County	29,676	43.3%
ARKANSAS			
Conway County Hospital	Morrilton Conway County	19,151	6.7%
Conway Regional Medical Center	Conway Faulkner County	60,006	0.0%
Mercy Hospital/Turner Memorial	Ozark Franklin County	14,897	6.3%
Mercy Hospital of Scott County	Waldron Scott County	10,205	0.8%
CALIFORNIA			
Lassen Community Hospital	Susanville Lassen County	27,598	9.1%
St. Elizabeth Community Hospital	Red Bluff Tehama County	49,625	6.1%

Hospital	Location	County Population	% Catholic
COLORADO			
Centura Health-St. Thomas More Hospital and Progressive Care Center	Canon City Fremont County	32,273	4.0%
Mercy Medical Center	Durango La Plata County	32,284	12.4%
IDAHO			
Clearwater Valley Hospital	Orofino Clearwater County	8,505	3.7%
St. Benedict's Family Medical Center	Jerome Jerome County	15,138	14.0%
St. Joseph Regional Medical Center	Lewiston Nez Perce County	33,754	8.7%
ILLINOIS			
St. Anthony's Memorial Hospital	Effingham Effingham County	31,704	37.8%
St. James Hospital	Pontiac Livingston County	39,301	18.5%
IOWA			
Avera Holy Family Hospital	Estherville Emmett County	11,569	15.0%
North Iowa Mercy Health Center	Mason City Cerro Gordo County	46,733	16.3%
St. Joseph Community Hospital	New Hampton Chicksaw County	13,295	33.8%
St. Joseph's Mercy Hospital	Centerville Appanoose County	13,743	11.9%
KANSAS			
Mercy Health System of Kansas	Fort Scott Bourbon County	14,966	5.8%
St. Catherine Hospital	Garden City Finney County	33,070	19.8%

Hospital	Location	County Population	% Catholic
KENTUCKY			
Flaget Memorial Hospital	Bardstown Nelson County	29,710	30.2%
Marcum & Wallace Memorial Hospital	Irvine Estill County	14,614	0.4%
Marymount Medical Center	London Laurel County	43,438	0.9%
St. Claire Medical Center	Morehead Rowan County	20,353	1.2%
St. Elizabeth Grant County	Williamstown Grant County	15,515	3.3%
St. Elizabeth Medical Center	Convington Kenton County	142,031	27%
MICHIGAN			
Lee Memorial Hospital	Dowagiac Cass County	49,477	8.2%
Mercy Health Services North	Grayling Crawford County	12,260	9.4%
Mercy Hospital	Cadillac Wexford County	26,360	9.1%
St. Francis Hospital	Escanaba Delta County	37,780	38.5%
Tawas St. Joseph Hospital	Tawas City Iosco County	30,209	17.2%
MINNESOTA			
Lakewood Health Center	Baudette Lake of Woods County	4,076	12.3%
St. Francis Medical Center	Breckenridge Wilken County	7,516	24.5%
St. Francis Regional Medical Center	Shakopee Scott County	57,846	5.8%
St. Gabriel's Hospital	Little Falls Morrison County	29,604	58.5%

Hospital	Location	County Population	% Catholic
MINNESOTA *(continued)*			
St. Joseph's Hospital	Park Rapids Hubbard County	14,939	11.7%
St. Mary's Regional Health Center	Detroit Lakes Belker County	27,881	18.3%
MISSOURI			
Breech Medical Center	Lebanon Laclede County	27,158	3.5%
SSM Arcadia Valley Hospital	Pilot Knob Iron County	10,726	4.4%
St. Francis Hospital	Maryville Nodaway County	18,670	21.8%
MONTANA			
Benefis Healthcare	Great Falls Cascade County	77,691	15.7%
Holy Rosary Health Center	Miles City Custer County	11,697	17.5%
St. James Community Hospital	Butte Silver Bow County	33,941	33%
NEBRASKA			
Faith Regional Health Services	Norfolk Madison County	10,931	78.8%
Good Samaritan Hospital	Kearney Buffalo County	37,447	16.8%
Providence Medical Center	Wayne Wayne County	9,364	9.1%
St. Francis Medical Center	Grand Island Hall County	48,925	22%
St. Francis Memorial Hospital	West Point Cuming County	10,117	41.3%

Hospital	Location	County Population	% Catholic
NORTH DAKOTA			
Carrington Health Center	Carrington Foster County	3,983	24.1%
Mercy Hospital	Devils Lake Ramsey County	12,681	36.9%
Mercy Hospital	Valley City Barnes County	12,545	20.9%
Oakes Community Hospital	Oakes Dickey County	6,107	15.2%
St. Aloisius Medical Center	Harvey Wells County	5,864	28.2%
St. Andrew's Health Center	Bottineau Bottineau County	8,011	11.4%
OHIO			
Clermont Mercy Hospital	Batavia Clermont County	150,187	15.6%
Good Samaritan Medical Center	Zanesville Muskingum County	82,068	10.6%
Mercy Memorial Hospital	Urbana Champaign County	36,019	6.2%
Trinity Medical Center	Steubenville Jefferson County	80,298	22.8%
OKLAHOMA			
Mercy Memorial Health Center	Ardmore Carter County	42,919	4.4%
OREGON			
Holy Rosary Medical Center	Ontario Malheur County	26,038	9.9%
St. Elizabeth Health Services	Baker City Baker County	15,317	8.3%

Hospital	Location	County Population	% Catholic
SOUTH CAROLINA			
St. Eugene Community Hospital	Dillon Dillon County	29, 114	0.7%
SOUTH DAKOTA			
Avera Queen of Peace Hospital	Mitchell Davison County	17,503	32.0%
Avera St. Luke's Midland Regional Medical Center	Aberdeen Brown County	35,580	27.4%
Sacred Heart Health Services	Yankton Yankton County	19,252	28.2%
St. Bernard's Providence Hospital	Milbank Grant County	8,372	26.5%
St. Mary's Hospital	Pierre Hughes County	14,817	19.2%
TEXAS			
Burleson St. Joseph Regional Health Center	Caldwell Burleson County	13,625	11.0%
Cogdell Memorial Hospital	Snyder Scurry County	18,634	7.5%
Crosbyton Clinic Hospital	Crosbyton Crosby County	7,304	8.2%
Highland Lakes Medical Center	Burnet Burnet County	22,677	7.4%
Madison St. Joseph Health Center	Madisonville Madison	10,931	1.8%
Spohn Bee County Hospital	Beeville Bee County	25,135	34.0%
Spohn Kleberg Memorial Hospital	Kingsville Kleberg County	30,274	50.1%
Swisher Memorial Hospital	Tulia Swisher County	8,133	17.2%

Hospital	Location	County Population	% Catholic
TEXAS *(continued)*			
Trinity Community Medical Center	Brenham Washington County	26,154	11.5%
Yoakum County Hospital	Denver City Yoakum	8,786	15.9%
VERMONT			
Fletcher Allen Health Care	Burlington Chittenden County	131,761	33.2%
VIRGINIA			
Bon Secours Maryview Medical Center	Portsmouth City Portsmouth	514,000	3.8%
WASHINGTON			
Our Lady of Lourdes Health Center	Pasco Franklin County	37,473	15.2%
St. Joseph's Hospital	Bellingham Whatcom County	127,780	8.0%
WEST VIRGINIA			
St. Joseph's Hospital	Buckhannon Upshur County	22,867	2.7%
WISCONSIN			
Langlade Memorial Hospital	Antigo Langlade County	19,505	45.2%
The Monroe Clinic	Monroe Green County	30,339	16.3%
St. Mary's Hospital Ozaukee	Mequon Ozaukee County	72,831	35.1%
St. Mary's Hospital	Rhinelander Oneida County	31,679	17.8%
St. Mary's Hospital of Superior	Superior Douglas County	41,758	20.6%

Hospital	Location	County Population	% Catholic
WISCONSIN *(continued)*			
St. Mary's Kewaunee Area Memorial Hospital	Kewaunee Kewaunee County	18,878	72.4%
St. Michael's Hospital	Stevens Point Portage County	61,405	53.5%

TOTAL Catholic Sole Providers in 1998: 91

TOTAL Catholic Sole Providers in 1997: 76**

** Total for 1997 is from *When Catholic and Non-Catholic Hospitals Merge: Reproductive Health Compromised* (Washington: Catholics for a Free Choice, 1998). Data as of July 1, 1997.

Sources: Hospitals identified as Catholic are those listed in the *Catholic Healthcare in the U.S.A Directory*, an on-line directory compiled by the Catholic Health Association (see CHA website: www.chausa.org/). The list of sole providers (as of July 1, 1998) is by the Health Care Financing Administration of the Department of Health and Human Services ("Providers of Services," at the agency's website: www.hcfa.gov/). County population is from *The 1990 Census of Population; General Population Characteristics* (US Bureau of the Census). Catholic population in each county is derived from *Churches and Church Membership in the United States, 1990* (Atlanta, GA: Glenmary Research Center, 1992).

Appendix G: Provision of Emergency Contraception in Catholic Emergency Rooms

Hospitals are listed alphabetically by name within each state. Bolded hospitals are sole providers.

			Hospital denies EC			
Hospital	Policy permits EC	No policy exists	Total	Provides referral w/number	Provides referral w/o number	Provides no referral
ALABAMA						
Mercy Medical, Daphne			x			x
Providence Hospital, Mobile			x			x
St. Vincent's Hospital, Birmingham			x			x
ALASKA						
Ketchikan General Hospital, Ketchikan			x			x
Providence Alaska Medical Center, Anchorage			x			x
Providence Kodiak Island Medical Center, Kodiak		x				
Providence Seward Medical Center, Seward			x			x
ARIZONA						
Carondelet Holy Cross Hospital, Nogales			x		x	
Carondelet St. Joseph's Hospital, Tucson			x		x	
Carondelet St. Mary's Hospital, Tucson			x		x	
St. Joseph's Hospital & Medical Ctr., Phoenix			x			x
ARKANSAS						
Conway County Hospital, Morrilton			x		x	
Conway Regional Medical Center, Conway			x	x		
Mercy Hospital & Pinewood Nursing Home, Waldron			x			x
Mercy Hospital-Turner Memorial, Ozark			x		x	
St. Bernard's Regional Medical Center, Jonesboro			x	x		
St. Edward Mercy Medical Center, Fort Smith			x		x	
St. Joseph's Regional Health Center, Hot Springs			x			x
St. Mary-Rogers Memorial Hospital, Rogers			x	x		
St. Vincent Infirmary Medical Center, Little Rock			x		x	
CALIFORNIA						
Alexian Brothers Hospital, San Jose			x	x		
Citrus Valley Medical Center, West Covina (Queen of the Valley Campus)			x	x		

Hospital	Policy permits EC	No policy exists	Hospital denies EC: Total	Provides referral w/number	Provides referral w/o number	Provides no referral
Daniel Freeman Marina Hospital, Marina Del Rey			x			x
Daniel Freeman Memorial Hospital, Inglewood			x	x		
Dominican Santa Cruz Hospital, Santa Cruz			x		x	
Lassen Community Hospital, Susanville			**x**			**x**
Little Company of Mary Hospital, Torrance			x	x		
Marian Medical Center, Santa Maria			x			x
Mercy American River Hospital, Carmichael (Mercy American River Campus)			x		x	
Mercy American River Hospital, Carmichael (San Juan Campus)			x	x		
Mercy General Hospital, Sacramento			x		x	
Mercy Hospital, Bakersfield			x	x		
Mercy Hospital of Folsom, Folsom			x	x		
Mercy Hospital & Health Services, Merced			x		x	
Mercy Medical Center, Redding			x	x		
Mercy Medical Center Mount Shasta, Mount Shasta			x		x	
Mercy Southwest Hospital, Bakersfield			x		x	
Mission Hospital Regional Medical Center, Mission Viejo			x		x	
O'Connor Hospital, San Jose		x				
Providence St. Joseph Medical Center, Burbank		x				
Queen of Angels, Hollywood Presbyterian Medical Center, Los Angeles			x			
Queen of the Valley Hospital, Napa			x			x
Petaluma Valley Hospital, Petaluma			x			x
Providence Holy Cross Medical Center, Mission Hills			x		x	
Redwood Memorial Hospital, Fortuna			x	x		
Robert F. Kennedy Medical Center, Hawthorne			x	x		
San Pedro Peninsula Hospital, San Pedro			x	x		
Santa Marta Hospital, Los Angeles			x	x		
Santa Rosa Memorial Hospital, Santa Rosa			x	x		
Santa Teresita Hospital, Duarte			x			x
Scripps Mercy Medical Center, San Diego		x				
Seton Medical Center, Daly City		x				
St. Agnes Medical Center, Fresno			x			x
St. Bernardine's Medical Center, San Bernardino			x			x
St. Dominic's Hospital, Manteca			x		x	
St. Elizabeth Community Hospital, Red Bluff			**x**	**x**		
St. Francis Medical Center, Lynwood		x				
St. Francis Medical Center of Santa Barbara, Santa Barbara			x	x		
St. John's Health Center, Santa Monica			x			x
St. John's Pleasant Valley Hospital, Camarillo			x	x		
St. John's Regional Medical Center, Oxnard			x			x
St. Joseph Hospital, Eureka		x				
St. Joseph Hospital, Orange			x			x
St. Joseph's Medical Center of Stockton, Stockton			x	x		

Hospital	Policy permits EC	No policy exists	Hospital denies EC: Total	Hospital denies EC: Provides referral w/number	Hospital denies EC: Provides referral w/o number	Hospital denies EC: Provides no referral
St. Jude Hospital, St. Jude Medical Center, Fullerton			x			x
St. Louise Hospital, Morgan Hill		x				
St. Mary Medical Center, Long Beach			x		x	
St. Mary Regional Medical Center, Apple Valley			x		x	
St. Mary's Medical Center, San Francisco			x		x	
St. Rose Hospital, Hayward			x		x	
St. Vincent Medical Center, Los Angeles			x		x	
COLORADO						
Centura Health-Mercy Medical Center, Durango			**x**		**x**	
Exempla/St. Joseph Hospital, Denver			x	x		
Penrose Community Hospital, Colorado Springs			x		x	
Penrose Hospital-St. Francis Health Services, Colorado Springs			x		x	
St. Anthony Hospital Central, Denver			x	x		
St. Anthony Hospital North, Westminster			x		x	
St. Francis Health Center, Colorado Springs			x		x	
St. Mary-Corwin Regional Medical Center, Pueblo		x				
St. Mary's Hospital & Medical Center, Grand Junction			x		x	
St. Thomas More Hospital & Progressive Care Center, Canon City	**x**					
CONNECTICUT						
Hospital of St. Raphael, New Haven			x		x	
St. Francis Hospital & Medical Center, Hartford (St. Francis Campus)		x				
St. Joseph Medical Center, Stamford		x				
St. Mary's Hospital, Waterbury			x	x		
St. Vincent's Medical Center, Bridgeport			x			x
DELAWARE						
St. Francis Hospital, Wilmington			x	x		
DISTRICT OF COLUMBIA						
Georgetown University Hospital			x		x	
Providence Hospital			x	x		
FLORIDA						
Bon Secours-St. Joseph Hospital, Port Charlotte			x	x		
Bon Secours-Venice Hospital, Venice		x				
Holy Cross Hospital, Fort Lauderdale			x	x		
Mercy Hospital, Miami			x		x	
Sacred Heart Hospital of Pensacola, Pensacola			x			x
St. Anthony's Hospital, St. Petersburg			x	x		

Hospital	Policy permits EC	No policy exists	Hospital denies EC: Total	Hospital denies EC: Provides referral w/number	Hospital denies EC: Provides referral w/o number	Hospital denies EC: Provides no referral
St. Joseph's Hospital, Tampa			x		x	
St. Joseph's Women's Hospital, Tampa			x		x	
St. Mary's Hospital, West Palm Beach			x		x	
St. Vincent's Medical Center, Jacksonville			x		x	
GEORGIA						
St. Joseph's Hospital of Atlanta, Atlanta			x		x	
St. Francis Hospital, Inc., Columbus			x		x	
St. Joseph Hospital, Augusta			x			x
St. Joseph's Hospital, Savannah			x		x	
St. Mary's Health Care System, Athens	x					
HAWAII						
St. Francis Medical Center West, Honolulu		x				
IDAHO						
Clearwater Valley Hospital, Orofino	**x**					
Mercy Medical Center, Nampa	x					
St. Alphonsus Regional Medical Center, Boise			x	x		
St. Benedict's Family Medical Center, Jerome			**x**			**x**
St. Joseph Regional Medical Center, Lewiston			**x**	**x**		
St. Mary's Hospital, Cottonwood			x		x	
ILLINOIS						
Alexian Brothers Medical Center, Elk Grove Village			x		x	
Columbus Hospital, Chicago			x			x
Good Samaritan Regional Health Center, Mt. Vernon			x	x		
Holy Cross Hospital, Chicago	x					
Holy Family Medical Center, Des Plaines			x	x		
Little Company of Mary Hospital & Health Care Centers, Evergreen Park			x			x
Loyola University Medical Center-Foster G. McGraw Hospital, Maywood			x			x
Mercy Hospital & Medical Center, Chicago			x	x		
Oak Park Hospital, Oak Park			x	x		
OSF St. Anthony Medical Center, Rockford			x			x
OSF St. James Hospital, Pontiac			**x**	**x**		
OSF St. Joseph Hospital, Belvidere			x		x	
Our Lady of Resurrection Medical Center, Chicago			x		x	
Provena Covenant Medical Center, Urbana			x	x		
Provena Mercy Center, Aurora			x			x
Provena St. Joseph Hospital, Elgin			x			x
Provena St. Joseph Medical Center, Joliet			x		x	
Provena St. Therese Medical Center, Waukegan			x			x

Hospital	Policy permits EC	No policy exists	Hospital denies EC: Total	Hospital denies EC: Provides referral w/number	Hospital denies EC: Provides referral w/o number	Hospital denies EC: Provides no referral
Provena St. Mary's Hospital, Kankakee	x					
Provena United Samaritans Medical Center-Logan Campus, Danville	x					
Provena United Samaritans Medical Center-Sager Campus, Danville	x					
Resurrection Medical Center, Chicago			x	x		
St. Anthony Hospital, Chicago			x	x		
St. Anthony's Health Center, Alton			**x**	**x**		
St. Anthony's Memorial Hospital, Effingham			x		x	
St. Bernard Hospital & Health Care Center, Chicago	x					
St. Clare's Hospital, Alton			x	x		
St. Clemet Hospital, Red Bud			x		x	
St. Elizabeth Medical Center, Granite City		x				
St. Elizabeth's Hospital, Bellevilles	x					
St. Elizabeth's Hospital of Chicago, Chicago	x					
St. Francis Hospital, Litchfield			x	x		
St. Francis Hospital & Health Center, Blue Island			x	x		
St. Francis Hospital of Evanston, Evanston			x	x		
St. Francis Medical Center, Peoria			x		x	
St. John's Hospital, Springfield	x					
St. Joseph Hospital, Chicago	x					
St. Joseph Medical Center, Bloomington			x	x		
St. Joseph Memorial Hospital, Murphysboro			x	x		
St. Joseph's Hospital, Breese		x				
St. Joseph's Hospital, Highland		x				
St. Margaret's Hospital, Spring Valley			x		x	
St. Mary Medical Center, Galesburg			x	x		
St. Mary of Nazareth Hospital Center, Chicago			x		x	
St. Mary's Hospital, Centralia			x			x
St. Mary's Hospital, Decatur	x					
St. Mary's Hospital, East St. Louis			x			x
St. Mary's Hospital, Streator			x	x		
INDIANA						
Memorial Hospital & Health Care Center, Jasper			x		x	
St. Anthony Medical Center, Crown Point			x		x	
St. Anthony Memorial Center, Michigan City			x	x		
St. Catherine Hospital of East Chicago, East Chicago			x		x	
St. Elizabeth Ann Seton Hospital, Boonville			x	x		
St. Elizabeth Medical Center, Lafayette			x		x	
St. Francis Hospital & Health Centers, Beech Grove			x		x	
St. John's Health System/St. John's Medical Center, Anderson			x		x	
St. Joseph Community Hospital, Mishawaka		x				

Hospital	Policy permits EC	No policy exists	Hospital denies EC: Total	Hospital denies EC: Provides referral w/number	Hospital denies EC: Provides referral w/o number	Hospital denies EC: Provides no referral
St. Joseph Hospital & Health Center, Kokomo			x		x	
St. Joseph's Regional Medical Center, Plymouth			x	x		
St. Joseph's Regional Medical Center, South Bend		x				
St. Margaret Mercy Healthcare Centers-North Campus, Hammond			x		x	
St. Margaret Mercy Healthcare Centers-South Campus, Dyer			x		x	
St. Mary's Medical Center, Hobart	x					
St. Mary's Medical Center of Evansville, Evansville		x				
St. Mary's Warrick, Boonville			x		x	
St. Vincent Carmel Hospital, Carmel			x	x		
St. Vincent Hospitals & Health Services, Indianapolis			x		x	
St. Vincent Mercy Hospital, Elwood	x					
St. Vincent New Hope, Indianapolis			x		x	
St. Vincent Williamsport, Williamsport			x	x		
IOWA						
Alegent Health-Mercy Hospital, Council Bluffs			x			x
Avera Holy Family Health, Estherville			**x**	**x**		
Covenant Medical Center, Waterloo			x			x
Marian Health Center, Sioux City			x			x
Mercy Health Center-St. Mary's Unit, Dyersville			x	x		
Mercy Hospital, Corning			x			x
Mercy Hospital, Iowa City			x			x
Mercy Hospital Medical Center, Des Moines			x		x	
Mercy Hospital of Franciscan Sisters, Oelwein			x			x
Mercy Medical Center, Cedar Rapids			x	x		
North Iowa Mercy Health Center, Mason City			**x**		**x**	
Samaritan Health System, Clinton		x				
St. Joseph Community Hospital, New Hampton			**x**		**x**	
St. Joseph's Mercy Hospital, Centerville			**x**	**x**		
KANSAS						
Central Kansas Medical Center-St. Rose Campus, Great Bend		x				
Mercy Hospital, Fort Scott			**x**		**x**	
Mercy Hospital, Independence			x	x		
Mt. Carmel Medical Center, Pittsburgh			x			
Providence Medical Center, Kansas City			x		x	
St. John Hospital, Leavenworth	x					
St. Catherine Hospital, Garden City			**x**	**x**		
St. Francis Hospital & Medical Center, Topeka			x	x		
Via Christi Regional Medical Center-St. Francis Campus, Wichita			x		x	

			Hospital denies EC			
Hospital	**Policy permits EC**	**No policy exists**	**Total**	**Provides referral w/number**	**Provides referral w/o number**	**Provides no referral**
Via Christi Regional Medical Center-St. Joseph Campus, Wichita			x			x
KENTUCKY						
CARITAS Medical Center, Louisville			x		x	
Flaget Memorial Hospital, Bardstown			**x**		**x**	
Lourdes Hospital, Paducah			x		x	
Marcum & Wallace Memorial Hospital, Irvine			**x**	**x**		
Marymount Medical Center, London			**x**		**x**	
Our Lady of Bellefonte Hospital, Ashland			x		x	
Our Lady of the Way Hospital, Martin			x	x		
St. Claire Medical Center, Morehead			**x**			**x**
St. Elizabeth Grant County, Williamstown			**x**		**x**	
St. Elizabeth Medical Center-North, Covington			**x**			**x**
St. Joseph Hospital, Lexington			x		x	
LOUISIANA						
Our Lady of Lake Regional Medical Center, Baton Rouge			x		x	
Our Lady of Lourdes Regional Medical Center, Lafayette			x			x
Sisters of Charity Coushatta Health Care Center, Coushatta			x		x	
Sisters of Charity-Schumpert Health System, Shreveport			x		x	
Sisters of Charity-St. Patrick Hospital, Lake Charles			x		x	
St. Frances Cabrini Hospital, Alexandria			x		x	
St. Francis Medical Center, Monroe			x		x	
St. Patrick's Hospital, Monroe			x		x	
MAINE						
Mercy Hospital, Portland			x		x	
St. Joseph Hospital, Bangor	x					
St. Mary's Regional Medical Center, Lewiston			x		x	
MARYLAND						
Bon Secours Hospital, Baltimore			x		x	
Holy Cross Hospital of Silver Spring, Silver Spring			x			x
Liberty Medical Center, Baltimore			x	x		
Mercy Medical Center, Baltimore	x					
Sacred Heart Hospital, Cumberland	x					
St. Agnes HealthCare, Baltimore			x			x
St. Joseph Medical Center, Towson		x				
St. Luke Institute, Silver Spring			x	x		
The Good Samaritan Hospital of Maryland, Baltimore			x	x		

Hospital	Policy permits EC	No policy exists	Hospital denies EC: Total	Hospital denies EC: Provides referral w/number	Hospital denies EC: Provides referral w/o number	Hospital denies EC: Provides no referral
MASSACHUSETTS						
Caritas Norwood Hospital, Norwood			x		x	
Caritas Southwood Hospital, Norfolk			x		x	
Carney Hospital, Boston			x		x	
Good Samaritan Medical Center, Brockton			x		x	
Holy Family Hospital & Medical Center, Methuen			x			x
Mercy Hospital, Springfield			x		x	
St. Anne's Hospital Corp, Fall River			x		x	
Saints Memorial Medical Center, Lowell			x		x	
St. Elizabeth's Medical Center, Boston			x		x	
Youville Hospital & Rehabilitation Center, Cambridge			x			x
MICHIGAN						
Battle Creek Health System, Battle Creek			x			x
Bon Secours Hospital, Grosse Pointe		x				
Borgess Medical Center, Kalamazoo			x		x	
Community Hospital, Battle Creek			x			x
Genesys Regional Medical Center, Grand Blanc	x					
Holy Cross Hospital of Detroit, Detroit			x		x	
Lee Memorial Hospital, Dowagiac		**x**				
Leila Hospital, Battle Creek			x			x
McPherson Hospital, Howell			x			x
Mercy General Hospital Partners- Sherman Boulevard Campus, Muskegon			x		x	
Mercy Health Services North, Grayling			**x**	**x**		
Mercy Hospital, Cadillac			**x**	**x**		
Mercy Hospital, Detroit			x			x
Mercy Hospital, Port Huron			x	x		
Providence Hospital & Medical Centers, Southfield			x	x		
Saline Community Hospital, Saline		x				
St. Francis Hospital, Escanaba		**x**				
St. John Detroit Riverview Hospital, Detroit			x		x	
St. John Hospital & Medical Center, Detroit			x	x		
St. John Macomb Hospital, Warren			x	x		
St. John Oakland Hospital, Madison Heights	x					
St. John River District Hospital, East China		x				
St. Joseph Mercy Hospital, Ann Arbor	x					
St. Joseph Mercy-Oakland, Pontiac			x		x	
St. Joseph's Mercy-East, Mt. Clemens			x			x
St. Joseph's Mercy-West, Clinton Township			x		x	
St. Mary Hospital, Livonia	x					
St. Mary's Health Services, Grand Rapids			x		x	
St. Mary's Medical Center of Saginaw, Saginaw			x		x	
Tawas St. Joseph Hospital, Tawas City			**x**			**x**

Hospital	Policy permits EC	No policy exists	Hospital denies EC: Total	Hospital denies EC: Provides referral w/number	Hospital denies EC: Provides referral w/o number	Hospital denies EC: Provides no referral
MINNESOTA						
Divine Providence Health Center, Ivanhoe			x			x
Graceville Health Center, Graceville			x			x
HealthEast St. Joseph's Hospital, St. Paul			x		x	
LakeWood Health Center, Baudette	x					
Queen of Peace Hospital, New Prague	x					
Regina Medical Center, Hastings			x			x
South Suburban Medical Center, Farmington	x					
St. Cloud Hospital, St. Cloud			x		x	
St. Francis Medical Center, Breckenridge			x		x	
St. Francis Regional Medical Center, Shakopee			x			x
St. Gabriel's Hospital, Little Falls	x					
St. Joseph's Area Health Services, Park Rapids			x			x
St. Joseph's Medical Center, Brainerd			x	x		
St. Mary's Hospital, Rochester			x		x	
St. Mary's Medical Center, Duluth			x	x		
St. Mary's Regional Health Center, Detroit Lakes	x					
MISSISSIPPI						
St. Dominic/Jackson Memorial Hospital, Jackson			x			x
MISSOURI						
Alexian Brothers Hospital, St. Louis			x		x	
Breech Regional Medical Center, Lebanon			x		x	
St. Joseph Health Center, Kansas City			x			x
SSM Arcadia Valley Hospital, Pilot Knob			x	x		
SSM DePaul Health Center, Bridgeton			x		x	
SSM St. Joseph Health Center, St. Charles			x		x	
SSM St. Joseph Hospital of Kirkwood, St. Louis			x			x
SSM St. Joseph Hospital West, Lake St. Louis			x			x
SSM St. Mary's Health Center, St. Louis			x	x		
St. Anthony's Medical Center, St. Louis			x		x	
St. Francis Hospital, Mountain View	x					
St. Francis Hospital & Health Services, Maryville		x				
St. Francis Medical Center, Cape Girardeau			x	x		
St. John's Mercy Hospital, Washington			x		x	
St. John's Mercy Medical Center, St. Louis			x	x		
St. John's Regional Health Center, Springfield			x		x	
St. John's Regional Medical Center, Joplin			x		x	
St. Mary's Health Center, Jefferson City	x					
St. Mary's Hospital of Blue Springs, Blue Springs			x		x	

Hospital	Policy permits EC	No policy exists	Hospital denies EC: Total	Provides referral w/number	Provides referral w/o number	Provides no referral
MONTANA						
Benefis Healthcare, Great Falls			**x**	**x**		
Holy Rosary Health Center, Miles City			**x**	**x**		
St. Vincent Hospital & Health Center, Billings		x				
St. James Community Hospital, Butte			**x**		**x**	
St. Joseph Hospital, Polson			x		x	
St. Patrick Hospital, Missoula			x		x	
NEBRASKA						
Alegent Health-Bergan Mercy Medical Center, Omaha			x			x
Faith Regional Health Services-East Campus, Norfolk			**x**		**x**	
Good Samaritan Hospital Health System, Kearney			**x**		**x**	
Providence Medical Center, Wayne	**x**					
St. Anthony's Hospital, O'Neill			x	x		
St. Elizabeth Community Hospital, Lincoln			x			x
St. Francis Medical Center, Grand Island			x		x	
St. Francis Memorial Health Center, Grand Island			**x**			**x**
St. Francis Memorial Hospital, West Point			**x**			**x**
St. Mary's Hospital, Nebraska City			x			x
NEW HAMPSHIRE						
Catholic Medical Center, Manchester			x			x
St. Joseph Hospital & Trauma Center, Nashua			x			x
NEVADA						
St. Mary's Regional Medical Center, Reno			x		x	
St. Rose Dominican Hospital, Henderson			x		x	
NEW JERSEY						
Holy Name Hospital, Teaneck			x		x	
Our Lady of Lourdes Medical Center, Camden			x	x		
St. Clare's Hospital, Boonton Township			x		x	
St. Clare's Hospital, Denville			x	x		
St. Clare's Hospital, Dover		x				
St. Clare's Hospital, Sussex		x				
St. Elizabeth Hospital, Elizabeth			x	x		
St. Francis Hospital-Franciscan Health System of NJ, Jersey City			x			x
St. James Hospital of Newark, Newark			x	x		
St. Joseph's Hospital & Medical Center, Paterson			x			x
St. Mary's Hospital, Passaic			x		x	
St. Mary's Hospital-Franciscan Health System of NJ, Hoboken			x			x
St. Michael's Medical Center, Newark			x		x	
St. Peter's University Hospital & Health System, New Brunswick			x		x	

Hospital	Policy permits EC	No policy exists	Hospital denies EC: Total	Hospital denies EC: Provides referral w/number	Hospital denies EC: Provides referral w/o number	Hospital denies EC: Provides no referral
NEW MEXICO						
St. Joseph Northeast Heights Hospital, Albuquerque			x			x
St. Joseph Rehabilitation Hospital, Albuquerque			x			x
St. Joseph West Mesa Hospital, Albuquerque			x			x
NEW YORK						
Benedictine Hospital, Kingston	x					
Cabrini Medical Center, New York			x		x	
Florence D'Urso Pavilion, Bronx			x		x	
Good Samaritan Hospital, Suffern			x			x
Good Samaritan Hospital Medical Center, West Islip			x			x
Kenmore Mercy Hospital, Kenmore			x			x
Mary Immaculate Hospital, Jamaica			x			x
Mercy Community Hospital, Port Jervis			x		x	
Mercy Hospital of Buffalo, Buffalo	x					
Mercy Medical Center, Rockville Centre			x			x
Mount St. Mary's Hospital of Niagara Falls, Lewiston	x					
Our Lady of Lourdes Memorial Hospital, Binghamton			x			x
Our Lady of Mercy Medical Center-Florence D'Urso Pavilion, Bronx			x		x	
Our Lady of Victory Hospital, Lackawanna			x		x	
Seton Health System-St. Mary's Division, Troy	x					
Sisters of Charity Hospital of Buffalo, Buffalo			x		x	
St. Agnes Hospital, White Plains			x			x
St. Anthony Community Hospital, Warwick			x		x	
St. Clare's Hospital, Schenectady		x				
St. Clare's Hospital & Health Center, New York	x					
St. Elizabeth Medical Center, Utica			x			x
St. Francis Hospital, Beacon		x				
St. Francis Hospital, Poughkeepsie	x					
St. James Mercy Hospital, Hornell			x		x	
St. Jerome Hospital, Batavia		x				
St. John's Queens Hospital, Elmhurst			x			x
St. Joseph Hospital, Cheektowaga	x					
St. Joseph's Hospital, Elmira			x		x	
St. Joseph's Hospital, Flushing			x			x
St. Joseph's Hospital Health Center, Syracuse		x				
St. Mary's Hospital, Rochester			x		x	
St. Mary's Hospital at Amsterdam, Amsterdam		x				
St. Mary's Hospital of Brooklyn, Brooklyn			x	x		
St. Peters' Hospital, Albany			x		x	
St. Vincents Hospital & Medical Center, New York			x			x
St. Vincent's Medical Center of Richmond, Staten Island			x	x		

			Hospital denies EC			
Hospital	**Policy permits EC**	**No policy exists**	**Total**	**Provides referral w/number**	**Provides referral w/o number**	**Provides no referral**
NORTH CAROLINA						
St. Joseph of the Pines, Pinehurst			x			x
NORTH DAKOTA						
Carrington Health Center, Carrington		**x**				
Mercy Hospital, Devils Lake		**x**				
Mercy Hospital, Valley City			**x**			**x**
Mercy Medical Center, Williston			x			x
Oakes Community Hospital, Oakes			**x**			**x**
Presentation Medical Center, Rolla	x					
St. Aloisius Medical Center, Harvey			**x**		**x**	
St. Alexius Medical Center, Bismarck	x					
St. Andrew's Health Center, Bottineau			**x**			**x**
St. Ansgar's Health Center, Park River			x		x	
St. Joseph's Hospital & Health Center, Dickinson			x			x
OHIO						
Clermont Mercy Hospital, Batavia			**x**		**x**	
Community Health Partners, Lorain			x			x
Franciscan Hospital-Mt. Airy Campus, Cincinnati			x		x	
Franciscan Hospital-Western Hills Campus, Cincinnati			x			x
Franciscan Medical Center-Dayton Center, Dayton			x		x	
Good Samaritan Hospital, Cincinnati			x		x	
Good Samaritan Hospital, Dayton			x			x
Good Samaritan Medical Center, Zanesville			**x**		**x**	
Marymount Hospital, Garfield Heights			x		x	
Mercy Hospital, Hamilton		x				
Mercy Hospital of Fairfield, Fairfield			x		x	
Mercy Hospital of Tiffin, Tiffin			x	x		
Mercy Hospital of Willard, Willard		x				
Mercy Medical Center, Springfield			x			x
Mercy Memorial Hospital, Urbana	**x**					
Mount Carmel East Hospital, Columbus			x		x	
Mount Carmel Medical Center, Columbus	x					
Providence Hospital, Sandusky			x			x
Riverside Mercy Hospital, Toledo			x		x	
St. Ann's Hospital, Westerville			x			x
St. Charles Mercy Hospital, Oregon			x	x		
St. Elizabeth Health Center, Youngstown			x		x	
St. Joseph Health Center-Eastland Campus, Warren			x			x
St. Rita's Medical Center, Lima			x		x	
St. Vincent Mercy Medical Center, Toledo			x		x	
Trinity Health Systems, Steubenville			**x**	**x**		

			Hospital denies EC			
Hospital	**Policy permits EC**	**No policy exists**	**Total**	**Provides referral w/number**	**Provides referral w/o number**	**Provides no referral**
OKLAHOMA						
Broken Arrow Medical Center, Broken Arrow			x			x
Hillcrest Health Center, Oklahoma City		x				
Mercy Health Center, Oklahoma City			x		x	
Mercy Memorial Health Center, Ardmore			**x**			**x**
St. Anthony Hospital, Oklahoma City			x		x	
St. Francis Hospital, Tulsa			x		x	
St. John Medical Center, Tulsa			x		x	
St. Joseph Regional Medical Center of Northern Oklahoma, Ponca City			x		x	
St. Mary's Mercy Hospital, Enid			x	x		
OREGON						
Holy Rosary Medical Center, Ontario			x		x	
Mercy Medical Center, Roseburg			x		x	
Peace Harbor Hospital, Florence			x		x	
Providence Milwaukie Hospital, Milwaukie			x	x		
Providence Newberg Hospital, Newberg			x			x
Providence Portland Medical Center, Portland			x		x	
Providence Seaside Hospital, Seaside			x		x	
Providence St. Vincent Medical Center, Portland			x			x
Sacred Heart Medical Center, Eugene			x			x
St. Anthony Hospital, Pendleton		x				
St. Charles Medical Center, Bend		x				
St. Elizabeth Health Services, Baker City	**x**					
PENNSYLVANIA						
Bon Secours Holy Family Regional Health System, Altoona			x		x	
Divine Providence Hospital, Williamsport			x			x
Good Samaritan Medical Center, Johnstown			x			x
Good Samaritan Regional Medical Center, Pottsville			x		x	
Hazleton-St. Joseph Medical Center, Hazleton			x			x
Holy Redeemer Hospital & Medical Center, Meadowbrook			x			x
Holy Spirit Hospital, Camp Hill			x		x	
Jeannette District Memorial Hospital, Jeannette			x		x	
Marian Community Hospital, Carbondale			x			x
Mercy Fitzgerald, Darby			x		x	
Mercy Hospital, Scranton			x			x
Mercy Hospital, Wilkes-Barre			x			x
Mercy Hospital of Philadelphia, Philadelphia			x			x
Mercy Hospital of Pittsburgh, Pittsburgh			x		x	
Mercy Providence Hospital, Pittsburgh			x		x	
Muncy Valley Hospital, Muncy			x	x		

Hospital	Policy permits EC	No policy exists	Hospital denies EC: Total	Provides referral w/number	Provides referral w/o number	Provides no referral
Nazareth Hospital, Philadelphia			x	x		
Sacred Heart Hospital, Allentown			x	x		
St. Agnes Medical Center, Philadelphia			x	x		
St. Francis Central Hospital, Pittsburgh			x		x	
St. Francis Hospital of New Castle, New Castle			x		x	
St. Francis Medical Center, Pittsburgh			x		x	
St. John Vianney Hospital, Downingtown			x		x	
St. Joseph Hospital, Lancaster			x		x	
St Joseph Medical Center, Reading			x			x
St. Mary Medical Center, Langhorne			x		x	
St. Vincent Health Center, Erie			x			x
RHODE ISLAND						
Our Lady of Fatima Hospital, North Providence			x		x	
St. Joseph Hospital for Specialty Care, Providence			x		x	
SOUTH CAROLINA						
Bon Secours-St. Francis Xavier Hospital, Charleston			x		x	
St. Eugene Community Hospital, Dillon			**x**			**x**
St. Francis Hospital, Greenville			x		x	
St. Francis Women's Hospital, Greenville			x			x
SOUTH DAKOTA						
Avera McKennan Hospital, Sioux Falls			x			x
Avera Queen of Peace Health Services, Mitchell			**x**		**x**	
Avera St. Luke's, Aberdeen			**x**		**x**	
Sacred Heart Health Services, Yankton			**x**		**x**	
St. Benedict Health Center, Parkston			x		x	
St. Bernard's Providence Hospital, Milbank			**x**		**x**	
St. Mary's Heathcare Center, Pierre	x					
St. Mary's Hospital, Pierre	**x**					
TENNESSEE						
Memorial Hospital, Chattanooga			x	x		
St. Thomas Health Services, Nashville			x			x
St Mary's Health System, Knoxville	x					
TEXAS						
Baptist-St. Anthony's Health System, Amarillo			x		x	
Burleson St. Joseph Health Center, Caldwell			**x**			**x**
Cogdell Memorial Hospital, Snyder		**x**				
Crosbyton Clinic Hospital, Crosbyton	**x**					
Grimes St. Joseph Health Center, Navasota			x		x	
Highland Lakes Medical Center, Burnet			**x**			**x**

Hospital	Policy permits EC	No policy exists	Hospital denies EC			
			Total	Provides referral w/number	Provides referral w/o number	Provides no referral
Jasper Memorial Hospital, Jasper			x	x		
Madison St. Joseph Health Center, Madisonville			**x**			**x**
Mercy Regional Medical Center, Laredo			x		x	
Providence Health Center, Waco			x			x
Santa Rosa Hospital, San Antonio			x		x	
Seton East Community Health Center, Austin			x			x
Seton Medical Center, Austin		x				
Seton Northwest, Austin			x		x	
Seton South Community Health Center, Austin			x		x	
Spohn Bee County Hospital, Beeville			**x**			**x**
Spohn Hospital Shoreline, Corpus Christi			x		x	
Spohn Hospital South, Corpus Christi			x		x	
Spohn Kleberg Memorial Hospital, Kingsville			**x**		**x**	
Spohn Memorial Hospital, Corpus Christi			x			x
St. Elizabeth Hospital, Beaumont			x			x
St. John Hospital, Nassau Bay			x	x		
St. Joseph Hospital, Houston			x			x
St. Joseph's Hospital & Health Center, Paris			x			x
St. Joseph Regional Health Center, Bryan			x		x	
St. Mary Hospital of Port Arthur, Port Arthur			x			x
St. Mary of the Plains Hospital, Lubbock			x		x	
St. Michael Health Care Center, Texarkana			x	x		
St. Paul Medical Center, Dallas			x			x
Swisher Memorial Hospital, Tulia		**x**				
Trinity Medical Center, Brenham			**x**		**x**	
Trinity-Mother Frances Health System, Tyler			x	x		
United Regional Health Care System, Eleventh Street Campus, Wichita Falls			x		x	
Villa Rosa Hospital, San Antonio			x			x
Yoakum County Hospital, Denver City			**x**			**x**
VERMONT						
Fletcher Allen Health Care, Burlington	**x**					
VIRGINIA						
Bon Secours De Paul Medical Center, Norfolk			x		x	
Bon Secours Maryview Medical Center, Portsmouth			**x**	**x**		
Bon Secours Memorial Regional Medical Center, Mechanicsville			x		x	
Bon Secours-Richmond Community Hospital, Richmond			x			x
Bon Secours-St. Mary's Hospital, Richmond			x			x

Hospital	Policy permits EC	No policy exists	Hospital denies EC: Total	Provides referral w/number	Provides referral w/o number	Provides no referral
Bon Secours Stuart Circle Hospital, Richmond			x			x
Mary Immaculate Hospital, Newport News			x		x	
St. Mary's Hospital, Norton			x			x
WASHINGTON						
Deer Park Health Center & Hospital, Deer Park			x		x	
Holy Family Hospital, Spokane			x	x		
Mount Carmel Hospital, Colville			x		x	
Our Lady of Lourdes Health Center, Pasco			**x**	**x**		
PeaceHealth-St. John Medical Center, Longview			x			x
Providence Centralia Hospital, Centralia			x		x	
Providence General Medical Center, Everett		x				
Providence Pacific Clinic, Everett	x					
Providence Seattle Medical Center, Seattle		x				
Providence St. Peter Hospital, Olympia			x		x	
Providence Toppenish Hospital, Toppenish		x				
Providence Yakima Medical Center, Yakima			x		x	
Sacred Heart Medical Center, Spokane			x			x
St. Clare Hospital, Tacoma			x		x	
St. Francis Hospital, Federal Way			x		x	
St. Joseph Hospital, Bellingham			**x**		**x**	
St. Joseph Hospital, Chewelah			x		x	
St. Joseph Medical Center, Tacoma			x		x	
St. Mary Medical Center, Walla Walla		x				
WEST VIRGINIA						
St. Joseph's Hospital of Buckhannon, Buckhannon		**x**				
St. Mary's Hospital of Huntington, Huntington			x		x	
Wheeling Hospital, Wheeling			x		x	
WISCONSIN						
Elmbrook Memorial Hospital, Brookfield		x				
Franciscan Skemp Healthcare-Mayo Health System, Arcadia	x					
Franciscan Skemp Healthcare-Mayo Health System, La Crosse Campus Medical Center, La Crosse			x		x	
Franciscan Skemp Healthcare-Mayo Health System, Sparta			x			x
Good Samaritan Health Center of Merrill, Merrill			x	x		
Holy Family Hospital, New Richmond			x		x	
Holy Family Memorial Medical Center, Manitowoc			x		x	
Langlade Memorial Hospital, Antigo		**x**				
Mercy Medical Center of Oshkosh, Oshkosh			x			x
The Monroe Clinic, Monroe			**x**		**x**	

Hospital	Policy permits EC	No policy exists	Hospital denies EC: Total	Provides referral w/number	Provides referral w/o number	Provides no referral
Sacred Heart Hospital, Eau Claire			x		x	
Sacred Heart Hospital, Tomahawk		x				
St. Agnes Hospital, Fond du Lac		x				
St. Catherine's Hospital, Kenosha			x		x	
St. Clare Hospital & Health Services, Baraboo			x			x
St. Elizabeth Hospital, Appleton			x		x	
St. Francis Hospital, Milwaukee			x			x
St. Joseph's Hospital, Chippewa Falls			x		x	
St. Joseph's Hospital, Marshfield			x			x
St. Joseph's Hospital, Milwaukee			x		x	
St. Joseph's Memorial Hospital, Hillboro			x	x		
St. Mary Kewaunee Area Memorial Hospital, Kenaunee			**x**			**x**
St. Mary's Hospital Medical Center, Green Bay			x		x	
St. Mary's Hospital Medical Center, Madison			x		x	
St. Mary's Hospital Ozaukee, Mequon			**x**			**x**
St. Mary's Hospital, Rhinelander			**x**			**x**
St. Mary's Hospital of Milwaukee, Milwaukee			x		x	
St. Mary's Hospital of Superior, Superior	**x**					
St. Mary's Medical Center, Racine			x	x		
St. Michael Hospital, Milwaukee			x		x	
St. Michael's Hospital, Stevens Point			**x**		**x**	
St. Nicholas Hospital, Sheboygan			x	x		
St. Vincent Hospital, Green Bay			x		x	
Victory Medical Center, Stanley			x		x	
Waupun Memorial Hospital, Waupan	x					
TOTALS	**55**	**53**	**481**	**106**	**225**	**149**

Number of Hospitals Called: 589

Further Information

Further information on Mergers is available from the following organizations:

Abortion Access Project of Massachusetts
552 Massachusetts Avenue
Suite 215
Cambridge, MA 02139
Phone: (617) 661-1161
Fax: (617) 492-1915
Email: info@repro-activist.org

California Women's Law Center
3460 Wilshire Boulevard
Suite 1102
Los Angeles, CA 90010
Phone: (213) 637-9900
Fax: (213) 637-9909
Email: cwlc@cwlc.org

Center for Reproductive Law and Policy
120 Wall Street, 18th Floor
New York, New York 10005
Phone: (212) 514-5534
Fax: (212) 514-5538
Email: info@crlp.org

MergerWatch, FPA
17 Elk Street
Albany, NY 12207
Phone: (518) 436-8408
Fax: (518) 436-0004
Email: info@mergerwatch.org

National Women's Law Center
11 Dupont Circle NW
Suite 800
Washington, DC 20036
Phone: (202) 588-5180
Fax: (202) 588-5185

Reproductive Freedom Project, ACLU
125 Broad Street, 18th Floor
New York, NY 10004
Phone: (212) 549-2633
Fax: (212) 549-2652
Email: rfp@aclu.org

Further information on Emergency Contraception is available from the following organizations:

The Alan Guttmacher Institute
1120 Connecticut Avenue NW
Suite 460
Washington, DC 20036
Phone: (202) 296-4012
Fax: (202) 223-5756
Email: policyinfo@agi-usa.org

The California Hospital Abortion Access Project
330 Townsen Street
Suite 204
San Francisco, CA 94107
Tel: (415) 546-7211
Fax: (414) 546-7634
Email: caral@aol.com

The Emergency Contraception Homepage
Operated by the Office of Population Research at Princeton University
www.opr.princeton.edu/ec/ecp.html

Physicians for Reproductive Health and Choice
1780 Broadway
10th Floor
New York, NY 10019
Tel: (212) 765-2322
Fax: (212) 246-5134
Email: PRCH@aol.com

The Population Council
One Dag Hammarskjold Plaza,
New York, NY 10017
Tel: (212) 339-0500
Fax: (212) 755-6052
pubinfo@popcouncil.org

Program for Appropriate Technology in Health (PATH)
4 Nickerson Street
Seattle
WA 98109
Tel: (206) 285-3500
Fax: (206) 285-6619
Email: info@path.org

Notes